Computer Vision
and Robotics in
Perioperative Process

Series in Computer Vision

ISSN: 2010-2143

Series Editor: C H Chen *(University of Massachusetts Dartmouth, USA)*

In recent years, there has been significant progress in computer vision in theory and methodology and enormous advancement on the application front, accompanied by rapid progress in vision systems and technology.

It is hoped that this book series in computer vision can capture most of the important and recent progress and results in computer vision. The target audiences cover researchers, engineers, scientists and professionals in many disciplines including computer science and engineering, mathematics, physics, biology, and medical areas, etc.

- Topics include (but not limited to)
- Computer vision theory and methodology (algorithms)
- Computer vision applications in biometrics, biomedicine, etc biometrics, biomedicine, etc
- Robotic vision
- New vision sensors, software and hardware systems and technology

Published

Forthcoming

Series in Computer Vision - Vol.5

Computer Vision and Robotics in Perioperative Process

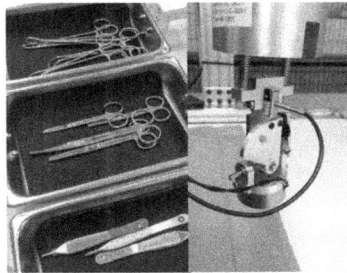

Yi Xu
JD.com Silicon Valley Research Center, USA

Huan Tan
GE Global Research, USA

Ying Mao
Dreamworld USA, Inc., USA

Lynn-Ann DeRose
GE Global Research, USA

World Scientific

NEW JERSEY · LONDON · SINGAPORE · BEIJING · SHANGHAI · HONG KONG · TAIPEI · CHENNAI · TOKYO

Published by

World Scientific Publishing Co. Pte. Ltd.
5 Toh Tuck Link, Singapore 596224
USA office: 27 Warren Street, Suite 401-402, Hackensack, NJ 07601
UK office: 57 Shelton Street, Covent Garden, London WC2H 9HE

British Library Cataloguing-in-Publication Data
A catalogue record for this book is available from the British Library.

Series in Computer Vision — Vol. 5
COMPUTER VISION AND ROBOTICS IN PERIOPERATIVE PROCESS
Copyright © 2018 by World Scientific Publishing Co. Pte. Ltd.

ISBN 978-981-3233-27-0

For any available supplementary material, please visit
http://www.worldscientific.com/worldscibooks/10.1142/10797#t=suppl

Preface

In early 2011, the United States Department of Veterans Affairs (VA) Innovation Initiative (VAi2) launched its second Industry Innovation Competition focused on leveraging the best ideas from the private sector. One of the new topics of this competition was to "fully automate sterilization of medical equipment." A team from GE Global Research, General Electric's research arm, responded to the competition and submitted a proposal titled "Automated Integrated Perioperative Process."

The team was managed by Lynn DeRose and consisted members from various research laboratories of GE Global Research with expertise in auto-ID, robotics, computer vision, mechatronics, business systems, and integrated system architecture. GE proposed to integrate these technologies in an innovative way to automate the sterile processing facility at VA. solution. The proposed solution was aiming to address safety concerns to patients that result from inadequately sterilized surgical implements. The integrated solution included automated implement recognition; automated kit building; automated kit transport and delivery; electronic validation of sterilization to support accountability; and data analytics to optimize inventory, operating room schedules, patient turn around, and other business processes.

The proposal was well-received by the VA. In 2012, GE Global Research was rewarded 2.5 million dollars by the VA to carry out the project. From 2012 to 2014, the GE team worked hard on research and development of the project. In summer 2014, GE demonstrated the integrated system successfully at VA's Community Living Center (CLC) at Orlando, Florida. In addition to the system demonstration, the research performed by the team also generated 6 publications in IEEE conference and journals, 1 granted patent and a few pending patent applications.

This research monograph provides a complete review of our multi-agent robotic system and its individual components. Algorithms and methods of each individual components are presented in great details. Insights and thoughts about the system and future commercialization strategy are also provided.

Yi Xu, Huan Tan, Ying Mao, and Lynn DeRose

Acknowledgments

This work was generously sponsored by the U.S. Department of Veterans Affairs Center for Innovation (VACI). Contract number was VA118-12-C-0051. The authors would like to thank Chuck Brown, Project Manager and Awilda Ramirez, Head of Sterile Processing for their help during the process of the project.

The high quality research resulted in peer-reviewed publications in IEEE journals and conferences. The authors would also like to thank Xianqiao Tong, Weston B. Griffin, Balajee Kannan, Viktor Holovashchenko, and Christopher Reardon, all of whom are co-authors of these publications, for their contributions to the research. In addition, the authors would like to thank Brandon Good, Bradford Miller, Dave Toledano and Dave Horney for their effort and contributions to the project.

Contents

List of Figures

List of Tables

Chapter 1

Automating the Perioperative Process

1.1 Background

The perioperative setting is the most resource intensive section of the hospital, accounting for about half of the hospitals budget. Any improvements in quality care and operational efficiency in the perioperative process would enhance the hospitals ability to meet budget targets. A hospital's perioperative department's performance also impacts patient safety. Approached systemically, patient throughput, surgical instrument identification and count, sterilization, and room turns can be dramatically improved.

On May 3, 2011, the standing Committee on Veterans Affairs in the United States House of Representatives held a hearing titled: "Sacred Obligation, Restoring Veteran Trust and Patient Safety." This hearing was initiated due to incidents of serious patient safety violations in VA medical facilities across the United States in Dayton, St. Louis, and Miami resulting in thousands of veterans across the country receiving notification of their potential risk for infectious diseases like the human immunodeficiency virus (HIV) and hepatitis.

The sterilization issues were mainly attributed to ineffective sterilization of reusable medical equipment (e.g., ear, nose, and throat endoscopes). The causes for these lapses in sterilization include:

- Inadequately trained staff; failure to develop device-specific training requirements.
- Trained staff with potential lapses in performance.
- Number of devices and brand types currently used across the different facilities.
- Lack of quality control
- Lack of effective oversight

These lapses pose potential risks to the safety of veterans. Automating the sterilization process will reduce the extent of human involvement in the process, reducing potential safety risks.

1.2   Current Perioperative Process

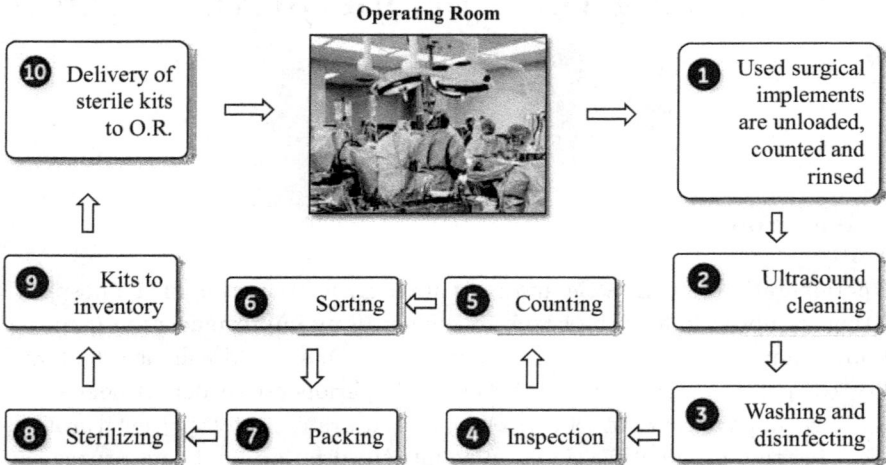

Fig. 1.1   The current perioperative process in VA medical facilities.

Fig. 1.1 shows the current steps of perioperative processing in VA medical facilities. The logistics of sterilizing, sorting, building, transporting, and counting sterile instruments is labor and capital intensive. Processing hundreds of types of instruments with very similar characteristics requires an extensive learning curve for hospital employees and perfect human diligence. Instruments and kits arrive in the dirty side of the sterilization room, where they are manually unloaded, counted, rinsed (Step 1). Then, they are cleaned in an ultrasonic cleaning system (Step 2). The washer/disinfector physically separates the dirty side of the sterilization room from the clean side (Step 3). The instruments are then removed from the washer/disinfector from the clean side, where they are inspected, counted, sorted, packed, and sterilized (Steps 48). The sterile kits are stored in inventory until needed (Step 9). The sterile kits are finally taken from inventory and delivered to the Operating Room (OR) (Step 10). The inventory and ORs are in a remote location from the sterilization room and may even be on a different floor of the hospital. The sterilization process directly affects the hospitals main profit center-the OR. Common mistakes made in the sterilization and delivery process such as incorrect kit constructs, counting errors, broken instruments, and un-sterile equipment affect patient safety, scheduling, throughput, and capacity in the OR.

1.3 Our Goal

To address this problem, we proposed an integrated system solution. Robotics, conveyors, auto-ID, and computer vision technologies are integrated to perform the sterilization steps. With the automated sterilization and delivery process, our main goal is to achieve increased safety, improved perioperative throughput, and enhanced care quality.

1.3.1 *Increased Safety*

The primary benefit from this automated solution is the development of a less manual process that reduces errors in the process and sub-standard sterilized instruments. By reducing human handling, we will increase the safety of the patients.

1.3.2 *Improved Throughput*

This automated solution will also increase the efficiency in OR scheduling due to increased kit accuracy and reduction in instrument counting time. In addition, by integrating automatic instrument tracking, handling, and sterilization together in a systemic way, we will enable more instrument throughput while improving on overall performance such as correct delivery.

1.3.3 *Enhanced Care Quality*

By implementing our automated solution, we can increase hospital quality and budget performance through reduction in surgical infections. We can also increase hospital capacity by reducing infection rates that require longer in-patient stays and by reducing operation set-up and room turn-around time. In the long term, improved staff to patient ratio will also have a significant impact on the quality of the care.

1.4 Our Approach

Fig. 1.2 shows a diagram of our proposed automated, integrated sterilization and instrument delivery process. We decided to focus our efforts on the sterilization room because robots are already widely used in hospitals to transport clinical supplies. TUG, a delivering robot manufactured by Aethon [Aethon (2018)], was already used in 27 VA facilities at the time of project initiation. Thus, our process does not include either delivering dirty instruments from ORs to sterilization process nor delivering sterilized surgical kits to storage room.

Before our automated process starts, wire trays containing dirty surgical instruments are returned from ORs and placed on a cart. Then, these surgical instruments are sorted, counted, inspected, and washed on the dirty side of the sterilization room. Then, instruments are disinfected before entering into the clean side of the

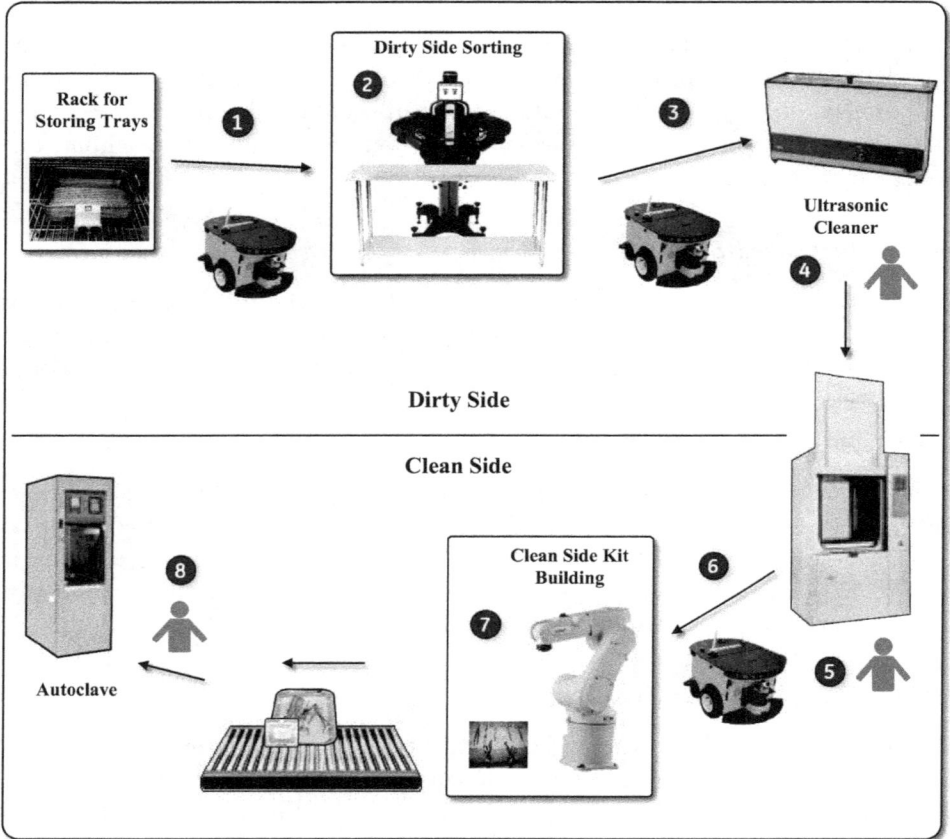

Fig. 1.2   Automated, integrated sterilization and delivery process. Among all the steps, steps 1, 2, 3,6, and 7 are performed by our robots. Steps 4, 5, 8 are performed by sterile processing nurses.

sterilization room. At the clean side, our robot places the surgical instruments into surgical kits based on the requests logged in the information management system. Finally the surgical kits are wrapped and placed into autoclave for sterilization. The remaining of this section discusses each step in more details.

1.4.1   *Move Dirty Instrument to Sorting Table - Step 1*

At the beginning of our automated process, the dirty surgical instruments are returned back from OR and randomly placed in instrument trays. The trays are then placed on a cart. We developed a mobile robotic system called TrayBot using an Adept Mobilrobots PowerBot [Adept Mobilerobots (2016)] equipped with a 6-DOF Schunk® PowerCube arm. We enhanced each tray with a customer designed han-

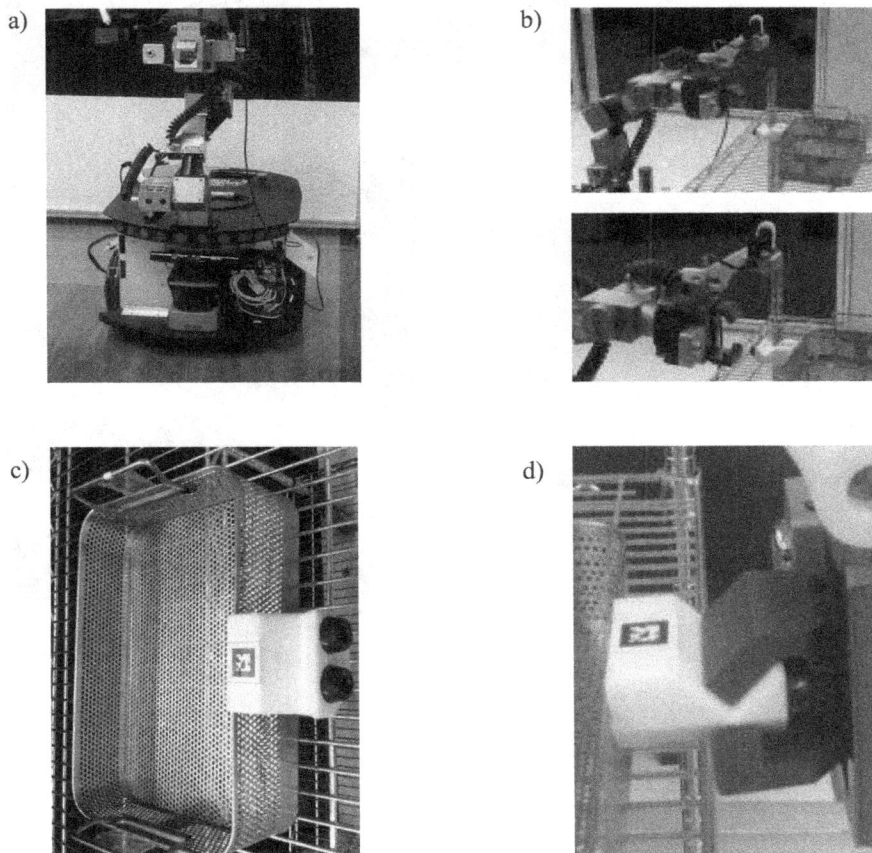

Fig. 1.3 a) Picture of our TrayBot. b) TrayBot reaches for a tray on the cart. c) Picture of a tray and its attachment with a 2D fiducial marker printed on it. d) TrayBot grasps the tray by the attachment using our self-aligning gripper.

dle. On top of the handle, there is a 2D fiducial marker, which serves as the ID of the tray. The down-looking camera on the PowerCube arm can detect the location and orientation of the fiducial marker. The tray can then be picked up by the arm using our customized end effector. TrayBot then navigates itself around the dirty side of the sterilization processing center and places the tray on the sorting table. Fig. 1.3 shows a picture of the Traybot, how Traybot approaches and picks up the dirty instrument tray, a picture of the tray with a handle, and how Traybot grasps the tray by the attachment.

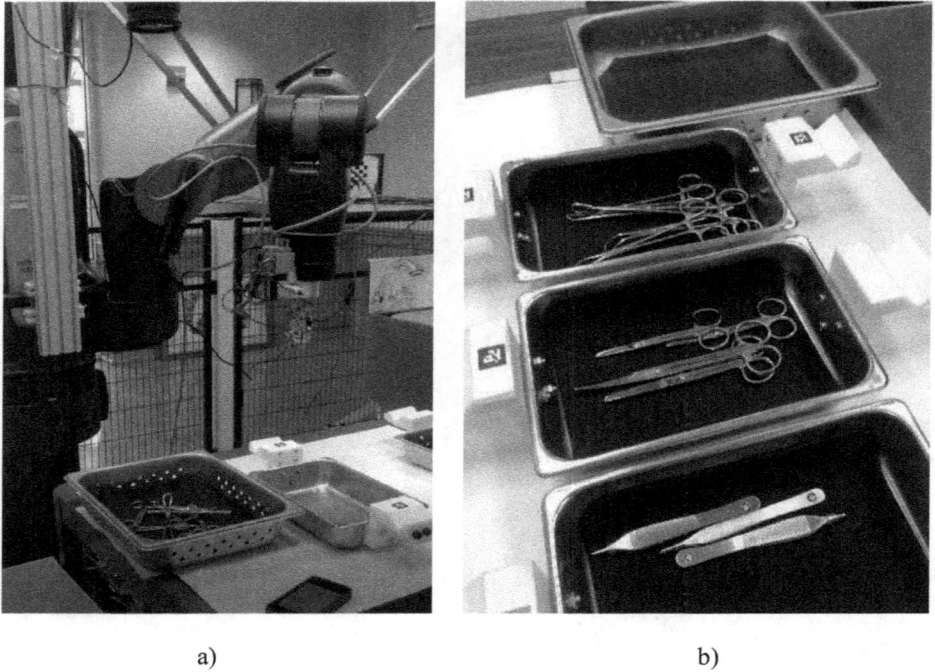

a)   b)

Fig. 1.4   a) A picture of Baxter sorting instruments from an unordered pile. b) The instruments are sorted into three trays based on their types by the Baxter.

1.4.2   *Sort the Instruments - Step 2*

After the dirty instrument trays are placed on the sorting table, they are sorted into separate trays based on their types (e.g., tweezers, scissors, etc.). This is to facilitate the ultrasonic washing step because different types of instruments require different scrubbing and washing procedures. Another purpose of this step is to identify each instrument and perform instrument tracking function. We developed a low cost sorting solution using a Baxter robot from RethinkRobotics® [Rethink Robotics (2018)]. The Baxter is equipped with a high definition camera for surgical instrument identification and pose estimation. A customer designed electromagnetic end effector is used pick and place the instruments.

Fig. 1.4 shows the a picture of Baxter and picture of the three sorted trays after sorting at the dirty side.

1.4.3   *Move Sorted Instruments to Cleaner - Step 3*

After Baxter sorts the dirty instruments into multiple trays based on instrument type, Traybot picks them up from the sorting table, navigates itself around the dirty side of the room, and places them on the working table of the ultrasonic cleaner for the sterile processing nurse to wash and disinfect the instruments.

1.4.4 *Wash and Disinfect Instruments - Step 4 & 5*

At this stage, a sterile processing nurse rinses the surgical instrument to remove any debris. Then the instruments are cleaned in the ultrasonic cleaner using a pre-determined procedure based on the type of the instruments. After cleaning, the trays are placed into the washer/disinfector. The specific wash cycle is loaded into the washer/disinfector. After the instruments are disinfected, they are ready to be processed further on the clean side of the sterile processing room. A second sterile processing nurse on the clean side fetches the trays from the washer/disinfector and places them on a table.

The main reason that a robot was not developed to perform operations on either side of the washer/disinfector is because with the advancement of Internet of Things, washer/disinfector will become connected with other devices and information management systems in a hospital. Thus, automating the washer/disinfector will become much easier. A robot that can push buttons or turn knobs will not be useful in the future.

1.4.5 *Move Cleaned Instruments to Kit Building Table - Step 6*

After cleaned instruments are fetched from washer/disinfector, the sterile processing nurse puts the trays on a table nearby. A second Traybot picks up the tray from the table, navigates itself around the clean side, and places them on the table of kit building robot.

1.4.6 *Build Surgical Kits - Step 7*

At this stage, the information management system informs the robot what kits to build and the list of surgical instruments of each list. In addition, the information management system also informs the robot the target location and orientation of each instrument within the kit tray. Then, the robot will pick up cleaned surgical instruments from the cluttered tray and place the instruments into empty kit trays. To achieve precision needed for this process, we use a clean room certified six-axis Adept® Viper S650 arm. Fig. 1.5 shows a picture of the Viper arm and a overhead high definition camera looking downward at the tray.

1.4.7 *Sterilization - Step 8*

The trays used for storing surgical kit are placed on a conveyor belt next to the table of the Viper arm. Once the robot completes the kit building task, it signals the information management system. Then, the system will turn on conveyor belt and move the kits to a station where it triggers an IR sensor, which will turn the conveyor belt off. The information management system will signal a dispenser

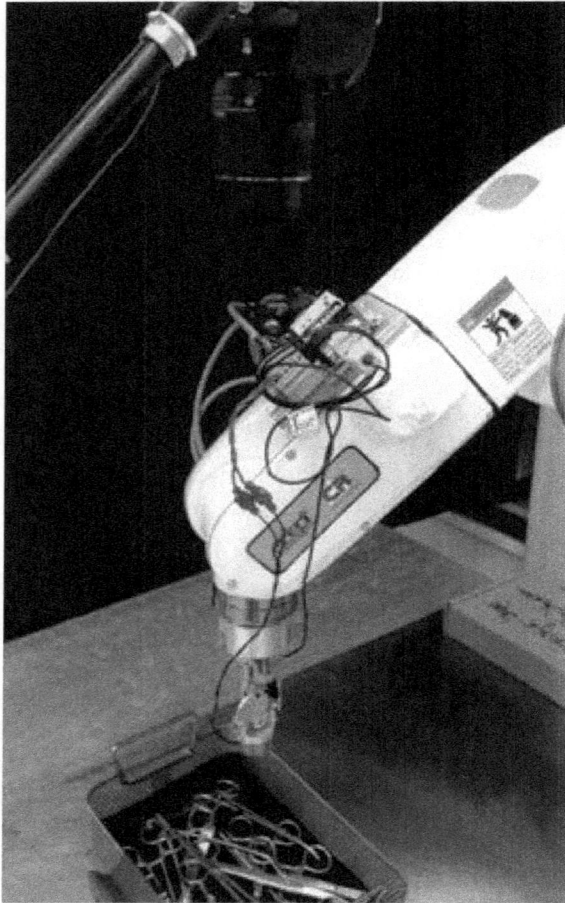

Fig. 1.5 A picture of the Adept® Viper s650 arm and a overhead digital camera used for vision processing.

to automatically dispense a chemical indicator into the completed kit. A sterile processing nurse then picks up the kit and moves it to the inspection station to validate whether the kit was built correctly and places the filter paper inside and puts the lid on the kit. The nurse will then place the kit into the autoclave for sterilization.

When the nurse moves the kit from the conveyor, the belt is reactivated and it moves the next surgical kit from the kit building table; ensuring continuous processing of completed surgical kits.

1.5 Organization of the Rest of the Book

The rest of the book will be organized as follows:

- **Chapter 2** discusses our distributed robotic software architecture [Tan *et al.* (2015a)]. This layered architecture highlights human factors in the automation workflow to provide a flexible and robust human-knowledge-based supervision and control for safe, reliable, and automated process for the health care industry.

- **Chapter 3** discusses our TrayBot, an integrated robotic system for autonomously transporting reusable surgical instrument trays in the sterilization processing center of a hospital [Tan *et al.* (2016)]. TrayBot performs steps 1, 2 and 3 illustrated in Fig. 1.2.

- **Chapter 4** discusses a novel single-view computer vision algorithm that identifies the next instrument to grip from a cluttered pile [Xu *et al.* (2014)]. This algorithm provides the perception capability to the two sorting robots (Step 2 and 7 in Fig. 1.2) on both sides of the sterile processing center.

- **Chapter 5** discusses the technical details of the two instrument sorting robots, including our compliant electromagnetic gripper design that is capable of picking up the identified instrument [Xu *et al.* (2015); Tan *et al.* (2015b)].

- **Chapter 6** discusses a human detection-based cognitive system for robots to work in human-existing environment and keep the safety of humans [Reardon *et al.* (2015)]. This integrated system is implemented with perception, recognition, reasoning, decision-making, and action.

- **Chapter 7** presents final demonstration results and offers more discussions.

Chapter 2

Human-Supervisory Distributed Robotic System Architecture

This chapter describes a human-supervisory distributed robotic software architecture, which has been applied in our multi-agent robotic system to automate the daily and repeated sterilization process [Tan *et al.* (2015a)]. Each robot is considered as an independent agent to perform assigned tasks with its own capability and coordinate their operations with other robots to ensure that the main process of the workflow satisfy the overall operation requirements. This layered architecture highlights human factors in the automation workflow to provide a flexible and robust human-knowledge-based supervision and control for safe, reliable, and automated process for healthcare industry.

2.1 Introduction

Robots are expected to perform tasks autonomously and intelligently, which is particularly desirable in fields such as space exploration, cleaning floors, mowing lawns, waste water treatment and delivering goods and services. A high level of degree of autonomy requires a coordinated integrated design of hardware, software, architecture, and infrastructure. Typical examples of highly autonomous systems are Curiosity and Opportunity Mars Rovers. However, due to the current limitations of technologies, especially in situational awareness, environmental modeling, knowledge representation, etc., a fully autonomous robotic system still requires lots of work in the future. Researchers have proposed a large amount of approaches to enable robots the capability of autonomy. Yet, the applications, especially commercialized products, have been confined within a small range, for example, iRobot Roomba, Google Self-Driving Car, etc.

Develop and commercialize a single autonomous robot is not easy. When it comes to develop a group of coordinated autonomous robots, the difficulty increases largely. This requires much higher level autonomy implementation as well as complex behavior and task scheduling and coordination [Tan (2014)]. Safety is another important concern in such autonomous robotic systems.

Gradually, it is well accepted that since the dream of full autonomy of various robots and applications are not easily realized, it is reasonable to take human factor into consideration, i.e., put human in the loop. By utilizing current state-of-art technologies to implement certain degree of robotic autonomy and bringing planning and coordination skills of a human in to a complex system, we can largely accelerate the development and commercialization of robotic products.

Supervision from human operators is desired to improve system performance and handle occasional exceptions due to the uncertainties in the environment and the operation process.

The rest of the chapter is organized as follows: Section 2.2 discusses related work in robotic architectures. Section 2.3 explains the components in this system in details. Section 2.4 uses an example to illustrate how to apply our architectural design. Section 2.5 describes the experimental setup and the results. Finally, Section 2.6 summarizes the contribution and proposes the future work.

2.2 Related Work

Currently, system architectures for individual robots could be divided into the following categories: Reactive, Symbolic, Connectionist, Hybrid, and Distributed [Tan (2012)].

A Reactive robotic system takes the sensory information as input, generates corresponding behaviors or actions using a tightly coupled sensory-motor control system. A typical example is Subsumption [Brooks (1986)].

A Symbolic robotic system uses traditional Artificial Intelligent (AI) concepts to represent the information processing processes and generate desired behaviors accordingly. Typical examples include: ACT-R [Anderson and Lebiere (1998)], SOAR [Lehman *et al.* (1996)], EPIC [Kieras and Meyer (1997)], Chrest [Gobet *et al.* (2001)], and Clarion [Sun (2003)].

Connectionist architectures for robotic systems use Artificial Neural Network (ANN)-like mechanisms to map the sensory information and the actions. A typical example is CAP2 [Schneider (1999)].

In order to realize human-like cognitive processes for robots, researchers realized a over-simplified architecture cannot represent the complex cognitive activities in human brains. A hybrid architecture could take the advantage of Reactive, Symbolic, and Connectionist architectures and provide a more robust and flexible approach for robots. Typical examples include: ISAC [Tan and Liang (2011)][Tan (2013)], RCS [Albus and Barbera (2005)], CHIP [Shrobe *et al.* (2006)], and JACK [Winikoff (2005)].

2.3 Multi-Agent Software Architecture

The basic principles of our system are distributed and human-supervised.

2.3.1 *Overall Robotic System Architecture*

Fig. 2.1 shows the overall architecture of our robotic system, which consists of *Management System*, *Supervisory System*, and *Functional Agent System*.

The *Management System* is responsible for task planning and scheduling, and communicating with external systems to obtain useful information and update the system log information in the database.

All the *Agents* receive the task information from the *Management System* and perform desired tasks by planning behavior sequences independently and autonomously. In most situations, the system performs correctly without replying on the *Supervisory System*. However, in some situations, human supervision is desired and necessary to facilitate the overall process. Data and process status are continuously updated and displayed by the *Supervisory System* for human operators to observe. User interface is also provided for human operators to manipulate the whole process at certain levels. We will discuss the three systems in more details.

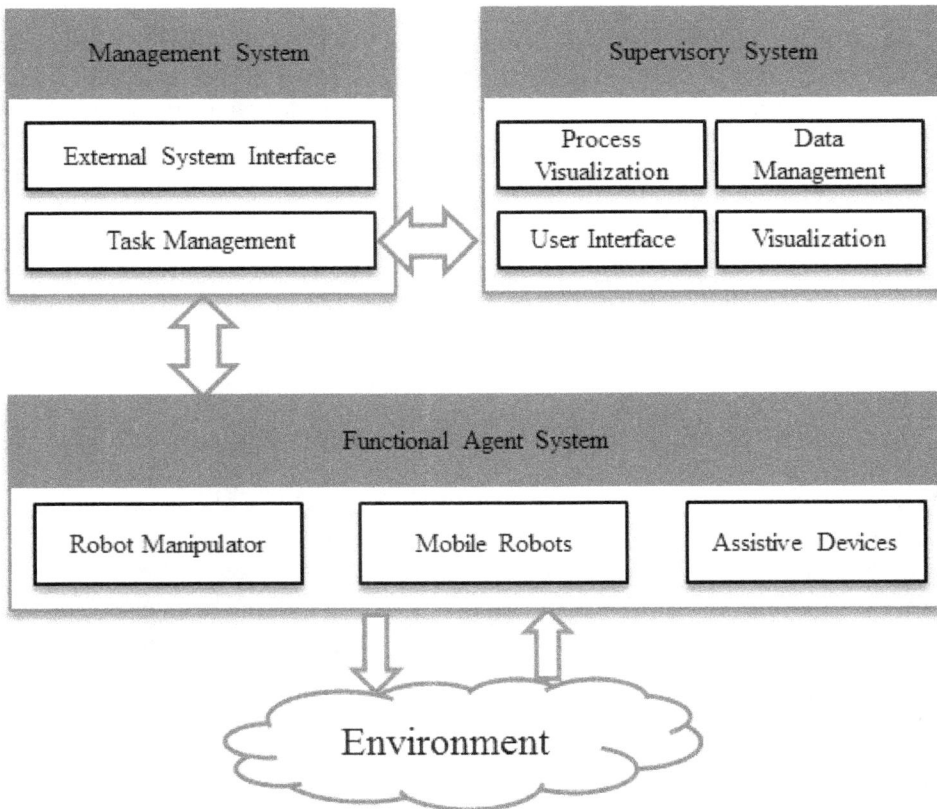

Fig. 2.1   A diagram of the overall system architecture.

2.3.1.1   *Management System*

The *Management System* consists of an *External System Interface* and a *Task Management* component.

The goal of providing an *External System Interface* is to increase the flexibility and robustness. With an external interface, the robot can communicate with external system. Once a central management system triggers the robot, the robot downloads task information from a sever. The task information and work logistics include goals, agents to be deployed, parameter settings, etc.

A task scheduling module, *Task Management*, is used to generate a sequence of task primitives to achieve the specific goal and assign the task primitives to each individual agent. Task primitives are scheduled and distributed to robots in the system according to different capabilities of the robots.

2.3.1.2   *Functional Agent System*

All the agents in the system have their own individual architectures to plan behavior sequences and reactively execute them chronically. The agents will continuously receive the updated planning information from the *Management system* and restart the planning process based on the information. We will explain these individual architectures in detail later in the Chapter.

2.3.1.3   *Supervisory System*

As stated earlier, we highlight the function of supervision from humans in our system. There are four major modules in the *Supervisory System*.

Process Visualization provides a description of the states of the overall system, which helps human operators to observe the operation of the system and provide necessary guidance or interference.

Using a *User Interface*, human operators can trigger the rescheduling process of the overall system. In our case, the rescheduling process is composed of modifying the sequence of the planned task primitives and enabling/disabling some task primitives. A human operator can easily modify the current task assignment and workflow of the system based on his/her judgment.

Device Visualization provides an intuitive description of the motions and status of all the robots and other assistive devices in the system. All the system information is stored in a *Data Management* system for human users to search, browse, track, and troubleshoot.

2.3.2   *Individual Robotic System Architecture*

Each agent should perform their assigned task independently and autonomously, which eventually affects the performance of the overall system. To achieve this goal, we designed a hybrid architecture for individual robot as shown in Fig. 2.2.

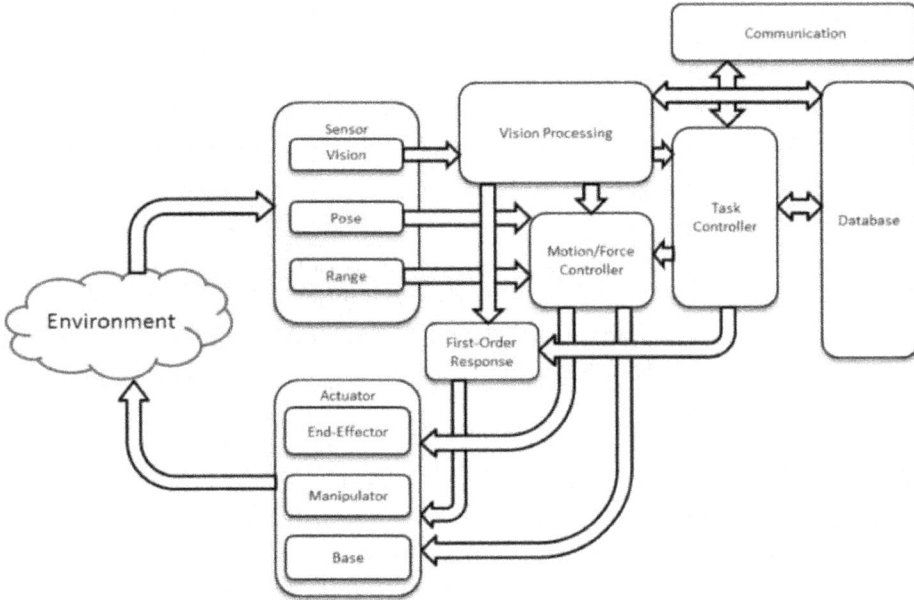

Fig. 2.2 A diagram showing individual robotic architecture.

2.3.2.1 *Communication*

Communication defines the communication protocols and interfaces between each individual robot and between robot and the *Management System*.

2.3.2.2 *Database*

The database is the memory component for the overall system, which stores required information for robots to use including localization, mapping, path planning, recognizing and identifying the types and positions of surgical tools, generating motion sequences composed of task primitives, etc.

2.3.2.3 *Task Controller*

The Task Controller sends out control signals to trigger different components directly and indirectly. There are two parts in this component: one is the task planning and scheduling, and the other is task monitoring and control, which are implemented using a *Finite State Machine* (FSM) and a *Decision Making Mechanism* (DMM) accordingly. Triggered by the commands received from the *Communication* interface, the *Task Controller* generates a sequence of task primitives for robots to execute.

2.3.2.4 *Sensors*

Sensors collect information from the environment and robot itself to reflect the current status of the system. Typical sensors include Lidar, camera, sonar, encoder, force/torque sensor, etc. The information obtained from such sensors are organized and published for robots to use.

2.3.2.5 *Actuators*

Actuators physically affect the environment and perform desired navigation and manipulation tasks using individual robot's capabilities. Normally, manipulation tasks use robotic manipulators as actuators; while navigation tasks use wheels as actuators to move the robot bases.

2.3.2.6 *Vision Processing*

Vision processing are implemented differently for robotic manipulators and mobile robots, but the common goal is to analyze vision information to provide labeled environmental information for robots to make decisions and to plan behaviors. In most robotic tasks, vision processing provides the pose of the object to be manipulated, the occupancy information of an environmental, and the landmark information for robotic localization, mapping, and navigation.

2.3.2.7 *Motion/Force Controller*

The *Motion Controller* drives the robot, including robot manipulators and mobile robots, to move to the desired goal positions [Tan *et al.* (2007)]. In this system, we implemented a simple proportionalintegralderivative (PID) controller to minimize the distance between the current robot configuration and the desired configuration. Motion control is realized by controlling the torques on the joints of the robots, which is done by the *Force Controller*.

2.3.2.8 *First-Order Response*

First-Order Response is a module making a decision significantly quickly to avoid any damage to the robot, the environment, and the devices. In a dynamic and unstructured environment, in order to meet the requirements of safety, robots should be able to make a low-level decision quickly and robustly to avoid any damage to the system and the environment.

2.4 Example of Implementation

Our motivation is to apply our proposed robotic architecture in VA hospitals. In our automated sterile processing, there are two stationary robots and two mobile robots involved in the overall system. Two mobile robots (TrayBots) are responsible

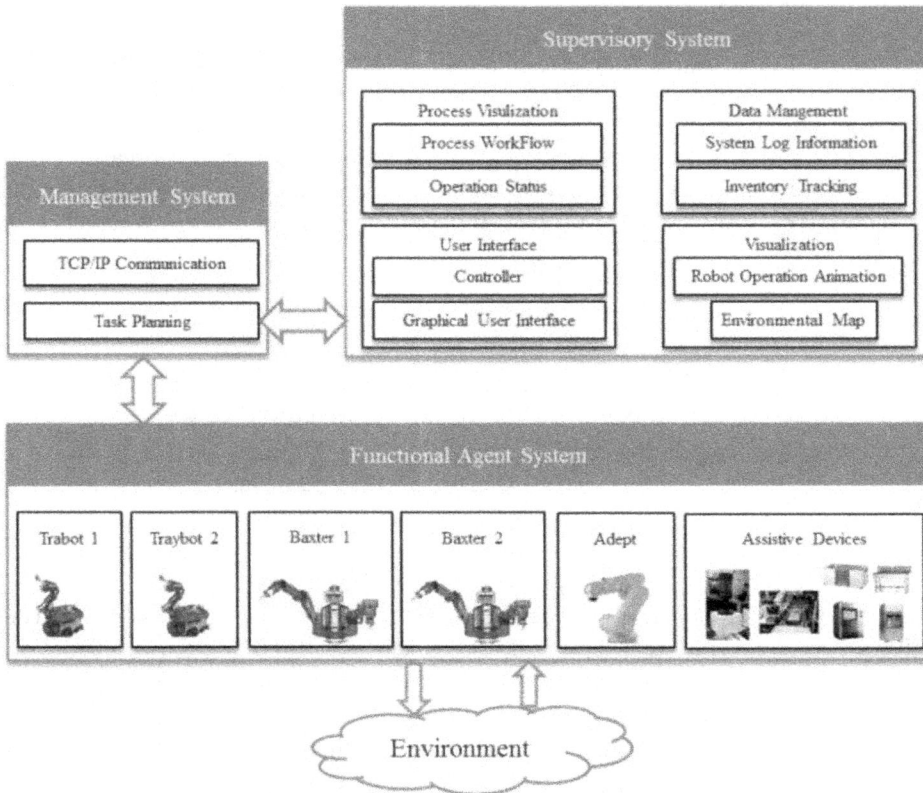

Fig. 2.3   Our implemented overall robotic architecture.

for transporting trays of surgical tools among working stations, one Baxter research robot performs sorting tasks, and the other Viper arm performs the kit-building task.

2.4.1   *Implemented Overall System Architecture*

Fig.2.3 displays an implemented overall system architecture.

2.4.1.1   *Management System*

The interface to the external systems is developed using TCP/IP communication. According to the daily requirements, the system assigns tasks to each robot and assistive device. The task assignment includes the desired goal of each task, related task parameters, and constraints on task sequences.

2.4.1.2 *Agent System*

For the transportation task, we develop our TrayBot using a PowerBot manufactured by Adept®. A 6-DOF Schunk® PowerCube arm is mounted on the surface of the robot for manipulation.

For the sorting tasks, the robots, used in our system is Baxter Research Robot produced by RethinkRobotics®. The assistive devices include LED lights for displaying system status, conveyor belt for transporting containers, sanitizer, sonicator, and auto-clave.

2.4.1.3 *Supervisory System*

In certain situations, human supervision is necessary to ensure that the overall system works correctly and follows the defined workflow. There are four major components for human operators to perform supervisory tasks.

Process workflow and operation status are displayed for human operators. After task planning, a task sequence is assembled and displayed on the screen. A task will be highlighted when the task is being executed. Meanwhile, an environmental map and the animations of robotic operations are visualized together. System log information and the tracked surgical tools are stored in the database for further analysis. Whenever a human operator determines that there are exceptions in the system, he/she can use a joystick controller to control the robots in the system, or modify the scheduled task sequence.

2.4.2 *Implemented Individual Robotic Architectures*

Since there are two types of robots in this system, the individual robotic architectures are also developed for these two types accordingly.

2.4.2.1 *Mobile Robot Architecture*

Given a task, the task controller generates a sequence of behaviors, which consists of waypoints for the robot to navigate through while taking obstacle avoidance into consideration.

Generated waypoints are sent to the *Motion Controller* to generate paths for robots to navigate and the potential field method is used to generate smooth paths. The range sensor in Fig. 2.2 is a laser sensor and a laser-based Simultaneous Localization and Mapping algorithm (SLAM) approach is applied to increase the precision of motion control. When arriving at the desired location on the waypoint sequence, the robot starts to search manipulation points in the environment using a camera, which is the vision sensor in Fig. 2.2.

After the manipulator is moved above the working station, the search task begins. A vision-based PID control algorithm is implemented for the manipulator. Database stores information about the environmental map and the trays. Communication is implemented using TCP/IP wireless method. The mobile robots obtain the task information from the *Management System*, and send the task status and system status information back to the *Management System*. The mobile robots also send information to the *Supervisory System* for visualization. Please refer to Chapter 3 "TrayBot: Transporting Surgical Tools in Hospitals" for a detailed discussion on the mobile robot architecture.

2.4.2.2 *Robotic Manipulator Architecture*

Vision processing component requires pre-computed templates created for each of the surgical tools. In the database, all the templates are stored as images of the edges of the surgical tools. When a new surgical tool is added, this database will need to be updated.

Since we are using a task primitive-based planning system, the database also stores basic task primitives: Start, Stop, Pause, Vision Processing, Returning, Moving-Up, Moving-Down, Moving-Forward, Moving-Backward, Moving-Left, Moving-Right, Reaching, Grasping, and Releasing.

Our vision processing system [Xu *et al.* (2014, 2015)] finds the location and orientation of the surgical tools in a tray and identifies which tool is on top of the pile. The grasping point is also identified using the vision processing algorithm. Please refer to Chapter 4 "Vision-based Instrument Singulation" for a detailed discussion on our vision processing algorithm.

The end effector is an electrical magnet gripper [Xu *et al.* (2014, 2015)], the current of which is modulated by a servomotor drive (Advanced Motion Controls® "Instrument Sorting Robots" for a detailed discussion on the end effector design and integration with Baxter robot and Viper arm.

2.5 Experimental Setup

We deployed our developed system in a laboratory environment. The experimental setup is shown in Fig. 2.4. The *Management System* and *Supervisory System are developed using* Java programming language. The Baxter Robot architecture and the Mobile Robot Architecture are developed on ROS-Fuerte platform using Python and C++ languages.

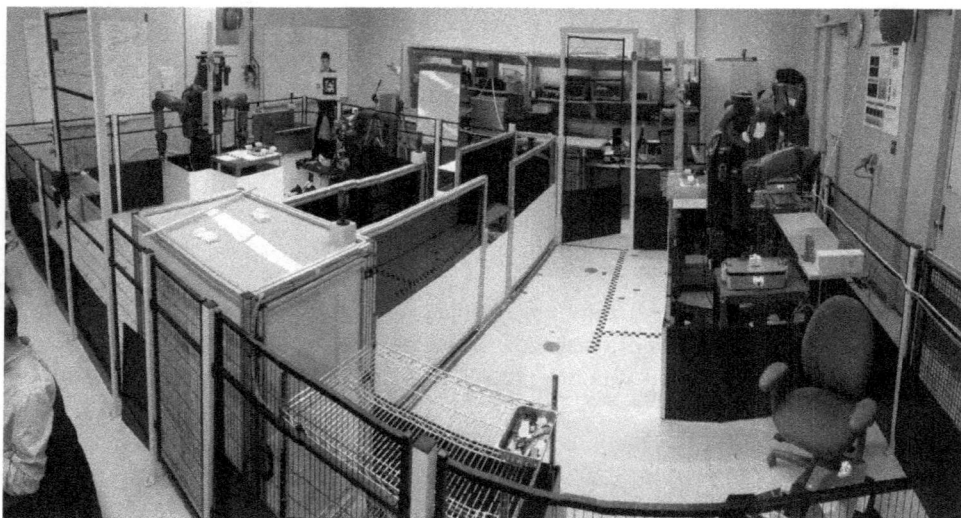

Fig. 2.4   Experimental setup in our lab.

Fig. 2.5 displays a typical tray picking-up sequence for the transportation scenario. The TrayBot moves to the cart (a), searched for the tray (b), then the robot plans the motion trajectory to reach the attachment of the try (c-d), and grab and hold the tray (e).

Fig. 2.6 displays a typical tray-placing sequence for the transportation task. The TrayBot moves to the working location (top), places the tray on the working table (middle), and moves the manipulator back to the home position (bottom).

Fig. 2.7 displays a typical sorting sequence for the Baxter robot in the system. The Baxter robot sorts the dirty surgical tools into corresponding trays for further cleaning. The Baxter robot uses a overhead downward looking camera. The system obtains and then analyzes the visual information on the operating table and computes the poses of the surgical tools to be grasped (top left). Then the Baxter robot moves its end effector to the top of the tray (top right), uses its electromagnetic gripper to grasp the tool (bottom left), and place the grasped tool in a designated tray based on its type (bottom right).

Quantitatively, the success rate of the transportation task is 100%. Our vision algorithm successfully locates the correct surgical tool for 95% of the time. The success rate of sorting is 80%, and the variation depends on the configuration of the tools in the tray. The success rate of the data transmission and information processing in the overall system is 100%.

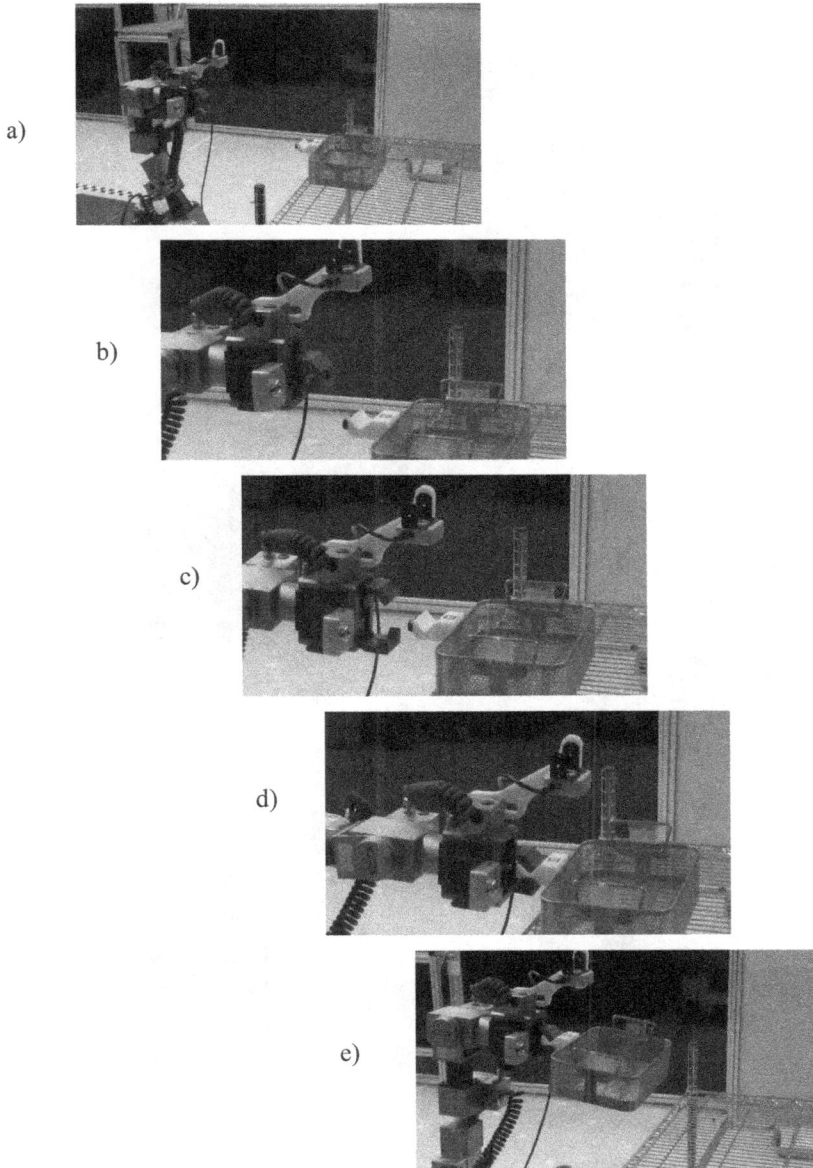

Fig. 2.5   Photo sequence showing a TrayBot picking-up a tray.

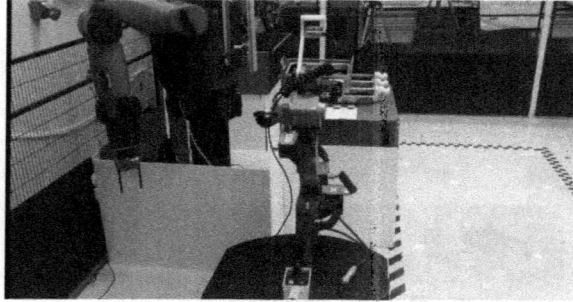

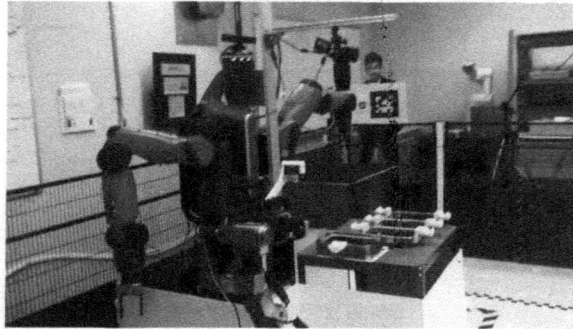

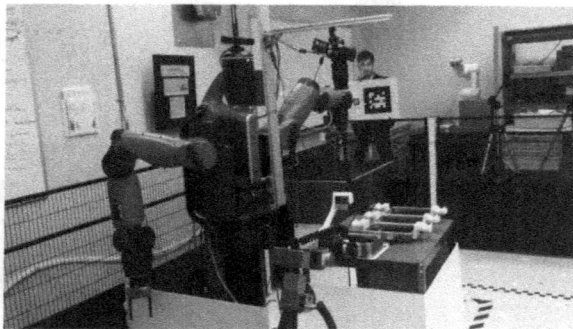

Fig. 2.6   Photo sequence of TrayBot placing a tray on the Baxter's table.

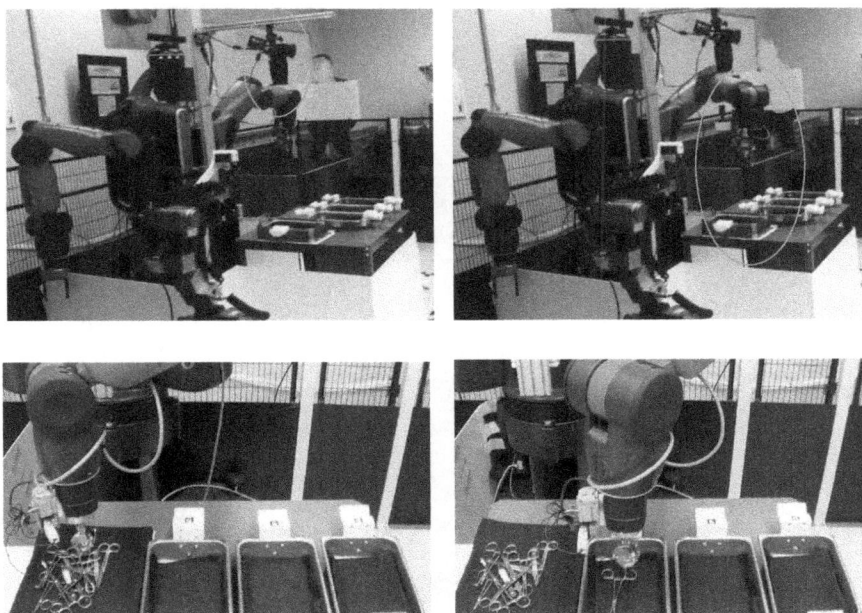

Fig. 2.7   Sequence of Baxter sorting surgical tools.

2.6 Summary and Future Work

This chapter describes a human supervisory system architecture for automating operation processes in healthcare industry. On the agent layer, each robot has its own individual architecture to perform tasks independently and autonomously. The system architecture has been tested and the experimental results satisfied the project requirements. In the future, we plan to improve the planning part in the system architecture to enable the capability of planning task sequences more flexibly and robustly.

Chapter 3

TrayBot: Transporting Surgical Tools in Hospitals

In this chapter, we detail a robust integrated system named TrayBot to autonomously perform manipulation of assets; specifically, transporting reusable surgical instrument trays in the sterile processing center of a hospital. Our method is based on a cognitive decision making mechanism that plans and coordinates the motions of the robot base and the robot manipulator at specific processing locations. A vision-based manipulator control algorithm is developed for the robot to reliably locate and subsequently pick up surgical tool trays. Furthermore, to compensate for perception and navigation errors, we developed a robust self-aligning end effector that allows for improved error-tolerance in larger workspaces.

3.1 Introduction

One of the key tasks throughout the sterilization process is to pick up trays of surgical instruments and transport them from one location to the other. For example, trays need to be picked up from counting stations and transported to the cleaning station. The pick-up task typically requires the robot to autonomously navigate to a location close enough for subsequent manipulation. Manipulation involves identification of the tray and visual-servoing the arm to the right position in space for the end effector to grasp the tray. We developed a mobile robot, called TrayBot, for this purpose.

Autonomous mobile robots with manipulation capabilities could enable increased flexibility in larger workspace and eliminate the need for multiple stationary robots to complete the same tasks. Therefore, we designed TrayBot for transporting trays that contain surgical instruments within a sterile processing center. Successful manipulation solutions for mobile robots need to overcome multiple challenges towards integrating navigation and manipulation capabilities. Mobility requires localization and navigation capability while avoiding collision of obstacles in the working environment [Choset (2005)]. Manipulation relies heavily on searching desired manipulation points, planning motion trajectories in high-dimensional task space, and grasping objects using end effectors [Lewis *et al.* (2003)]. In order to ensure robust operations, a tightly integrated design, which incorporates navigation and manipulation under increasing operational uncertainty, is required. Planning in navigation and manipulation should share information to increase the rate of successful object manipulation. However, errors due to noise and uncertainty make the manipulation tasks more difficult. Error for the navigation system is typically more significant than the manipulation system and this unbalanced error distribution desires algorithms that are capable of handling the errors at different levels and compensate the error in the final manipulation process.

The rest of this chapter is organized as follows: Section 3.2 discusses the related work in manipulation for mobile robots, vision-based control, and end effector design; Section 3.3 discusses designs of the hardware components. Section 3.4 introduces the architecture of the integrated system and explains the major modules and algorithms in the system; Section 3.5 focuses on the experimental setup and results; and Section 3.6 summarizes this chapter and proposes future work.

3.2 Related Work

Manipulation using mobile robots has recently attracted increased attention from the robotics community. Researchers proposed an amount of architectures and methods which identify perception, planning, and execution as three crucial issues for such manipulation tasks. An important feature of execution in manipulation using mobile robots is to integrate mobility and manipulation. Typical robots developed for mobile manipulation include: Willow Garage's PR2 [Willow Garage (2015)], DLR's Rollin' Justin [DLR (2016)], DFKI Robotics Innovation Center's AILA [DFKI (2018)], PowerBot [Adept Mobilerobots (2016)], Robotnaut [NASA Johnson Space Center (2016)], HERB [Srinivasa *et al.* (2010)] , etc.

An important technology for mobile manipulation is Simultaneous Localization and Mapping (SLAM) [Leonard and Durrant-Whyte (1991)], which solves the problem of constructing or updating a map of an environment while simultaneously keeping track of an agent's location within it. Klein and Murray proposed parallel tracking and mapping for small AR workspaces (PTAM) [Klein and Murray (2007)] to implement marker-less visual SLAM. Their major contribution is to perform tracking and mapping in parallel, allowing computationally-expensive optimization to be carried out in a batch fashion. Mur-Artal et al. proposed a system called ORB-SLAM [Mur-Artal *et al.* (2015)]. ORB-SLAM uses ORB features [Rublee *et al.* (2011)] for tracking and reconstruction of 3D map points within the environment. In addition to using only visual sensors, fusion with other sensors can often provide a better localization result [Kam *et al.* (1997)]. In our system, we use laser-based navigation and localization software which is part of the PowerBot platform.

Some researchers are interested in developing kinematic and dynamic control systems for mobile manipulation. Seraji proposed a unified approach, which treats the base nonholonomy and the kinematic redundancy in a unified manner to formulate new task constraints for mobile manipulators [Seraji (1998)]. Padois et.

al. presented a unified modeling framework for the reactive control of wheeled mobile manipulators, which is particularly well suited for handling complex tasks in dynamic environment [Padois *et al.* (2007)]. Since the working environment is designed to be well-structured, a cognitive decision making mechanism which plans and coordinates the motions of the robot base and the robot manipulator at specific processing locations is sufficient.

There has been growing interest on how a robot can perform complex grasping in unstructured environment. For example, Papazov et al. use a Kinect sensor to digitize a scene of household objects for robotic grasping [Papazov *et al.* (2012)]. PR2 utilizes a laser scanner for object manipulation [Chitta *et al.* (2012)]. Collet and Srinivasa proposed an approach that can recognize all objects in the scene and estimate their full pose based on learned models of the objects using SIFT descriptors [Collet *et al.* (2011)]. To improve detection, a multi-view approach with three cameras is used. Saxena et al. train a detector that can identify a few good picking points from more than two images [Saxena *et al.* (2008)]. Then, triangulation is used to obtain the 3D picking location. In our system, since we have the freedom to augment the surgical tool tray for easier manipulation, we only use one single camera mounted on the robot end effector to locate a fiducial marker on the attachment of the tray. The fiducial marker is correlated with the grasping point.

A well-designed robot gripper can increase success rate of manipulation tasks. A general guideline for gripper design was developed by Causey and Quinn [Causey and Quinn (1998)]. Self-aligned grippers are popular for their ability to enhance manipulation reliability. Zhang and Goldberg proposed a modular approach to design trapezoidal gripper jaws that push, topple and fix the part at the desired part orientation for standard parallel gripper [Zhang and Goldberg (2001)]. Sam and Nefi designed a flexible gripper for handling food products of various size and shape [Sam and Nefti (2008)]. We also designed a self-align gripper to handle the localization errors in order realize fast locating and grasping of surgical tool tray.

3.3 Hardware Component Design

Since we have the freedom to change or augment the components used in the sterile processing process, we designed a few things to enable efficient tray recognition, graping and transportation. In this section, we will discuss the design details.

Surgical instruments are placed in trays after being used in ORs and transported using a cart to the serial processing center. Fig. 3.1 (top) displays the cart used to transport trays. In our system, the height of the surface of the cart is 88cm, and the dimension of the surface of the cart is 90cm (L) x 60cm (W). The trays in our setup are 28cm (L) x 19cm (W) as shown in Fig. 3.1 (bottom). Trays will be placed on the cart without fixed locations and orientations. An attachment is mounted on each tray for robots to grasp. The attachment is also augmented with a visual fiducial marker for easy identification and localization.

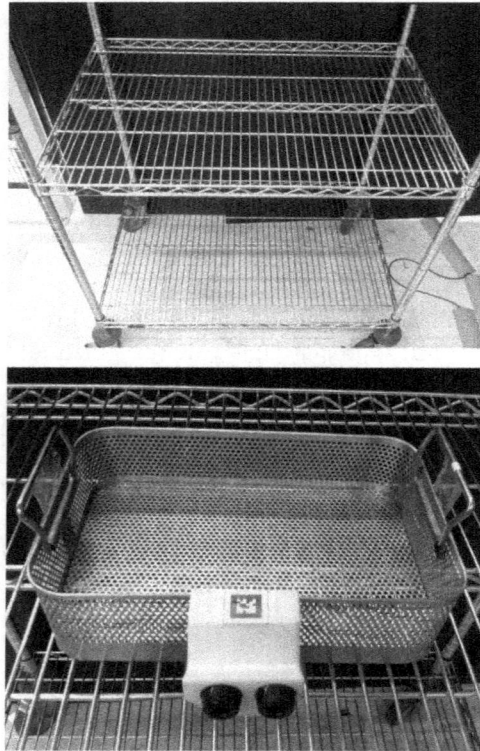

Fig. 3.1   Storage cart (top) and tray (bottom) used in our system.

The task requires the mobile robot to move to the cart and pick up a tray. Due to mechanical limitation of the PowerCube arm, the robot cannot reach every corner of the surface of the cart. According to the size of the tray used in our project, we calculated the manipulation area on the cart surface as shown in Fig. 3.2. The shaded area defines where the tray should be placed. In this area, trays could be placed with orientations within the limitation of the gripper. The desired working location is designed to allow 86cm between the center of the front wheel line and the edge of the cart, which translates to 56cm between the center of base of the manipulator and the edge of the cart.

The robot used in our system is a Pioneer 3 PowerBot manufactured by Adept®. A 6-DOF Schunk® PowerCube arm is mounted on the surface of the robot for manipulation as shown in Fig. 3.3 (top). We put a camera on the sixth link of the arm to fetch images from a top-down view of the manipulation area as shown in Fig. 3.3 (bottom image, top circle). The attached end effector is also shown in Fig. 3.3 (bottom image, bottom ellipse) is developed in our lab to handle errors generated from vision, locomotion, and manipulation. An attachment part is designed and attached to the tray. The jaws and the attachment have two sets of orthogonal

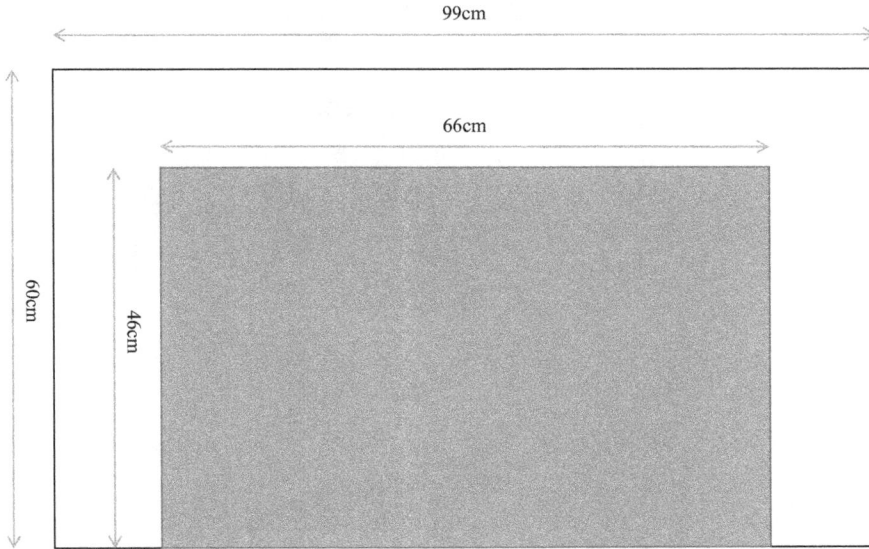

Fig. 3.2   Manipulation area on a cart.

slopes that self-aligns the tray relative to the arm with simple closure of the jaws. These are illustrated in Fig. 3.4. The slope features on the upper jaw and the upper part of the attachment aligns translation in the X plane. The slope features of the bottom jaw and the bottom part of the attachment part align translation in the Y plane. Full closure of the jaws constrains translation in the Z plane. The pitch, roll and yaw of the tray are also constrained by these slope features and the closure of the jaws.

The software system for the mobile robot runs on an on-board computer with Intel Core 2 CPU 4300 running at 1.8GHz. We use ROS Fuerte with Ubuntu 12.04 as our software platform.

3.4   Integrated System Design

In this section, we detail the architecture of the integrated system and explains the major modules and algorithms in the system.

3.4.1   *System Overview*

Fig. 3.5 displays the general system architecture used in for our TrayBot. The overall system is controlled by the *Task Planning* module, which plans all the activities in the robotic system.

Given a task, the system plans the waypoints for the robot to navigate through, taking obstacle avoidance into consideration. Generated waypoints are then sent

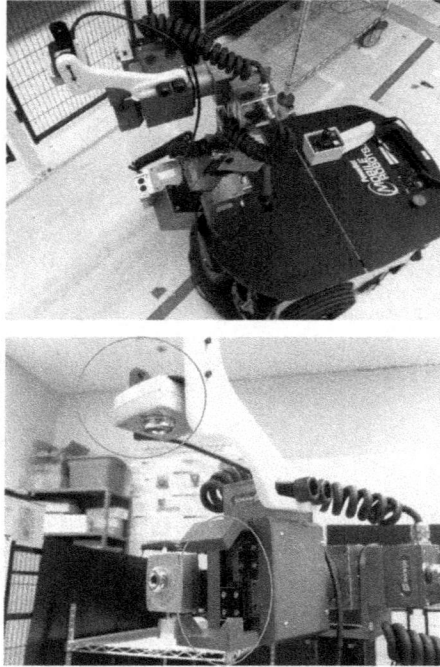

Fig. 3.3 Images showing the camera mounted on the arm. The top image shows a top down view of the Schunk® arm mounted on the Adept® PowerBot base. The bottom image shows the camera and the custom designed end effector.

to the *Task Planning* for validation. This validation process makes certain that collision with obstacles is avoided. In order to satisfy safety requirements, in any situation that a collision is unavoidable, the system defers the task. Successful validation of waypoints triggers the *Robot Base Motion Planning* module to generate paths for robots to navigate through the environment. Reactive obstacle avoidance is also included in the *Robot Base Motion Planning*. In this process, *Laser-based SLAM* is applied to increase the precision of localization.

After arriving at the desired location on the waypoints sequence near the tray storage cart, the TrayBot starts to search manipulation points in the environment. During the search task, TrayBot moves the manipulator above the cart surface and captures a sequence of images. Images obtained by the camera are processed to detect square fiducial markers. If found, the ID of the tray and the position and orientation of the square fiducial marker is sent to the *Task Planning* for decision making. If TrayBot cannot find a fiducial maker, *Task Planning* will generate a signal to inform human operators that the task failed.

Position and orientation data alone cannot guarantee that TrayBot can successfully grasp the tray in the environment and the *Task Planning* is responsible for

Side View   Front View

Schunk gripper module

Upper jaw

Tray attachment

Lower jaw

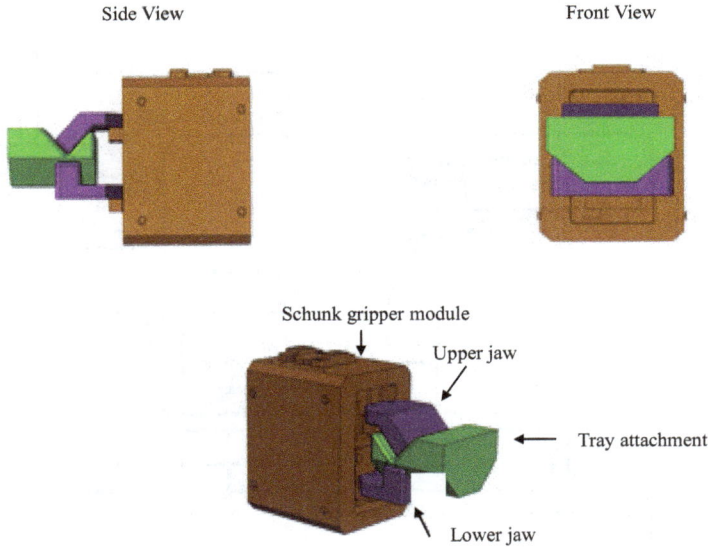

Fig. 3.4   Illustration of self-aligning gripping mechanism.

making a decision. The decision is based on the capability of the robot and the safety issues. For example, even the robot can see the object, it may not be able to perform the manipulation task due to mechanical limitations of the manipulator. The mobility of the robot base could increase the chances of completing a manipulation task since it has the ability to make minor positional adjustments. The *Task Planning* module decides whether the robot base needs to move in order to manipulate the object. If it is impossible for robot to manipulate the object even it can move someplace else, *Task Planning* module rejects the task.

After *Task Planning* module decides that a manipulation task is within the capability of the robot, it plans the motion trajectories for the robot base and the manipulator. Generated motion trajectories are sent to the *Navigation* and *Manipulation* to complete the task. In the rest of the Section 3.4 , each module is discussed in more details.

3.4.2   *Task Planning*

The *Task Planning* module is the crucial part that governs the system. It is important for robots to decide when to control the base or the arm to ensure successful task completion and minimize the energy consumption. Such a decision making process is based on incorporating fused sensory information from environment, robot, other robots. and prior knowledge. Thus, a cognitive decision making process is used to address the navigation and manipulation planning problem. Table 3.1 displays pseudo code of the task planning in our system.

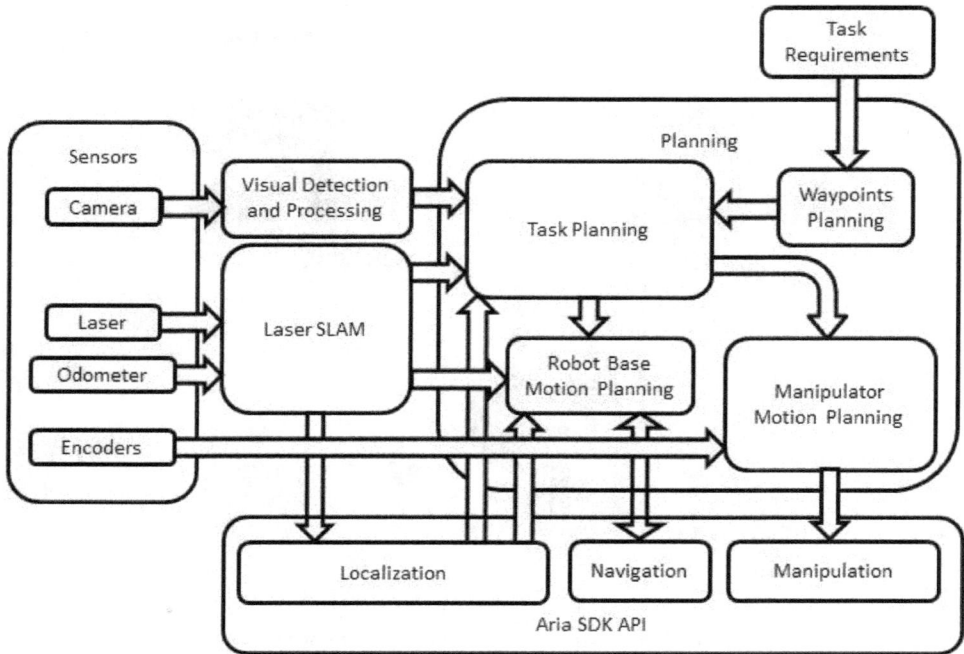

Fig. 3.5   Diagram of system architecture of our TrayBot.

At the navigation stage, triggered by *Task Planning*, *Waypoints Planning* generates a sequence of waypoints to facilitate manipulation tasks at working locations. After waypoints are generated and validated, *Task Planning* triggers the *Robot Base Motion Planning* to plan the motion trajectories of the robot base using Potential Field-based methods [Khatib (1986)]. This planning process provides a plan for the robot to navigate through all the planned waypoints and execute corresponding desired manipulation tasks at each processing location.

Once the robot arrives at one processing location, the robot needs to perform certain manipulation tasks, e.g., grasping. In the manipulation stage, there are two major sub-tasks for the robot: 1) ensure the grasping and picking-up of the tray; 2) minimize energy consumption. Thus, the planning strategy in manipulation stage is to move the robot base to increase the working space and the success rate of manipulation and optimize an energy consumption equation, for example, by moving the base a little bit, the robot can use less torque on its joints to perform manipulation tasks.

3.4.3   *Navigation and Localization*

Navigation of a robot base in the environment requires two parts of work: localization and motion control. In our system, we used a laser sensor to increase the precision of localization. Obstacle avoidance is implemented in our system by in-

Table 3.1 Pseudo code for task planning module

Repeat until all searching points are searched or object detected)

Move manipulator to the next search point

Detect object

if (object detected)

Optimize *Energy Consumption Cost Equation*

if (object within the desired manipulation area)

Compute manipulation point
Plan motion trajectories of the manipulator
Manipulate

else

Plan motion trajectories of the robot base
Move the base to new working location
Detect object

if (Object detected)

Compute manipulation point
Plan motion trajectories of the manipulator)
Manipulate

endif()
Move robot base to original working location

endif()

endif()

End

corporating a reactive Potential Field-based motion control method. For example, every time when the robot is within the movement from A to B and finds an obstacle on its movement path, it re-plan a path to avoid the obstacle.

3.4.4 *Vision-based Manipulator Control*

To enable the identification and localization of a tool tray placed on a cart, we place a chilitag on a small horizontal surface area of the attachment as shown in Fig. 3.6. A chilitag is a square shaped, black-white fiducial marker used in Augmented Reality applications [Bonnard *et al.* (2013)]. Each chilitag provides an ID of the tray. In addition, it also provides the location and orientation of the tray. A camera , which is mounted 15cm above the gripper, is used to detect chilitags. The camera is looking downward at the horizontal plane of the cart surface. Standard image

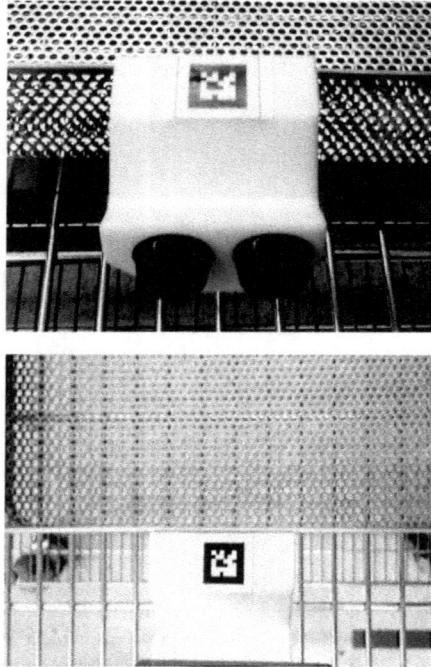

Fig. 3.6   (Top) Tray attachment with Chilitag printed on a flat surface. (Bottom) Top-down view from the camera mounted on end effector.

un-distortion is applied to correct for radial distortion before chilitag detection.

3.4.4.1   *Search for the Tray*

After the system notifies the presence of a tray with an ID, a searching strategy is used to find the desired chilitag in the working space. Due to limited length of the manipulator and the height of the mounted camera, we developed an M-step searching process. At each step, robot moves its end effector coupled with the camera from left to right or from right to left in N straight lines. These straight lines are distributed from near to far. On each line, L searching points are defined. At each searching point, TrayBot captures an image using the camera and determine whether the desired chilitag is present. After searching on N lines from left to right, if the desired chilitag is still not found, TrayBot moves its base forward with distance d and continues the searching on the next N straight lines. The geometry of these lines remains the same as in the previous step. A total of M steps are performed; resulting in searching at $MxNxP$ points in the worst case scenario. Fig. 3.7 shows an illustration of our searching strategy. After M-step searching, if the desired chilitag is still not found, the robot notifies human operators the failure. Otherwise, the robot computes the position and the orientation of the chilitag.

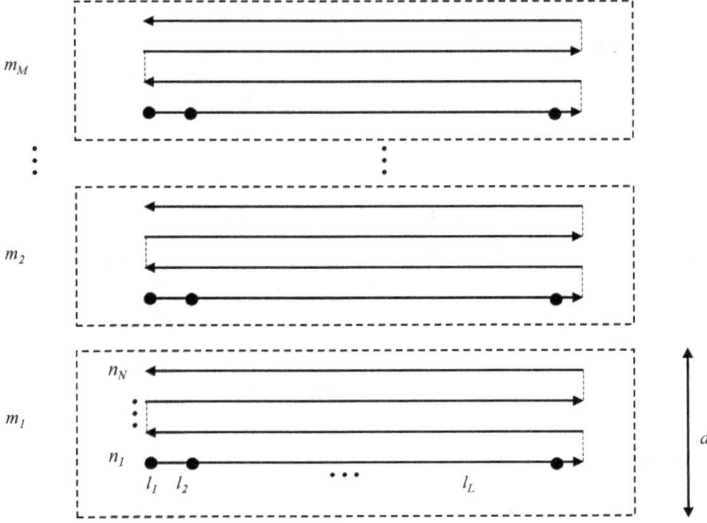

Fig. 3.7 Illustration of our M-step searching strategy.

3.4.4.2 *Determine the Manipulation Point*

At a calibration stage, we capture a frame using the camera at a configuration where the gripper is ready to fully grasp the tray attachment. We store the image coordinate of the center of the chilitag as a reference point C_0. During live operation, TrayBot captures a series of images until a chilitag is detected with its center at image coordinate C_1. Because the camera's image plane is parallel with the surface of the cart, a 2D translation is sufficient to bring the gripper to its target location for gripping. This translation vector T can be simply computed by $T=C_1$-C_0 . We then simply scale the translation T from image coordinates to world coordinates based on the real-world and observed dimension of the chilitag. The orientation of the chilitag could be computed using the detected chilitag four corners. The world coordinates of a chilitag reflects the position of a manipulation point.

If the manipulation point is too far from the base link, the manipulator will be stretched out too much. This results in instability of the control system and vibration at the end effector. If the manipulation point is too close to the base link, the failure rate of finding an inverse kinematic solution may increase. Thus, we constrain the manipulation point to be within a desired area.

To find the best motion of the manipulation and the robot base, We applied a decision making mechanism that utilizes the mobility of the robot. An energy consumption function is defined as in Eq. 3.1:

$$L = f(\mathbf{J}, \mathbf{Q}_J) + D^T \mathbf{Q}_d D \qquad (3.1)$$

where J is a 6-dimensional vector representing the joint angles of the robot arm, D is a displacement value that changes the distance between the robot base and the cart, and Q_J and Q_d are weight matrices. When the robot is at different locations by varying D, the desired kinematic configuration for grasping the attachment on a tray can be computed. We simplified our consumption function by deploying a linear equation as shown in Eq. 3.2:

$$L = \mathbf{J}^T \mathbf{Q}_J \mathbf{J} + D^T \mathbf{Q}_d D \tag{3.2}$$

By minimizing Eq. 3.2, a desired displacement motion distance can be computed as D. If D is smaller than a pre-defined threshold value D_{th}, the robot will move forward or backward with displacement D-D_{th}. If the robot moves its base, it needs to redo the searching process to find the world coordinates of the chilitag; if it does not need to move its base, it goes to the manipulation stage of the task.

3.4.4.3 *Grasp the Tray*

At the manipulation stage, the robot plans the motion trajectories of the end effector to manipulate the object. The motion planning should avoid any collision between the robot and the environment. Thus, we put two constraints on the motion planning: one is to avoid self-collision, and the other is to avoid collision with any objects in the environment.

3.5   Experimental Setup and Results

The proposed integrated navigation and manipulation system was validated. For the searching part, we choose $M = 2$, $N = 4$, and $L = 3$. The length of each of the N lines is 30cm each. The distance between each line is 5cm and we choose $d = 20cm$. These values were chosen because images obtained from the camera can cover up to $16cm$ wide area. Our parameter settings enable the robot to cover $50cm x 46cm$ area to satisfy the project requirements. For the manipulation planning in Section 3, we choose $D_{th} = 40cm$.

Based on the requirements described above, we design two experiments:

- Determine the success rate of the grasping manipulation of successful picking-up of the tray.
- Determine the maximum angle of the tray orientation that still allows the self-aligning gripper to successfully grasp the tray.

3.5.1   *Success Rate*

A tray was placed on the cart randomly within the manipulation area (Fig. 3.2 and at fixed orientation of $\theta = 0°$.

Fig. 3.8 displays the pictures obtained during one of the experimental runs. At the beginning, TrayBot moves to waypoint near the cart (a). TrayBot then searches

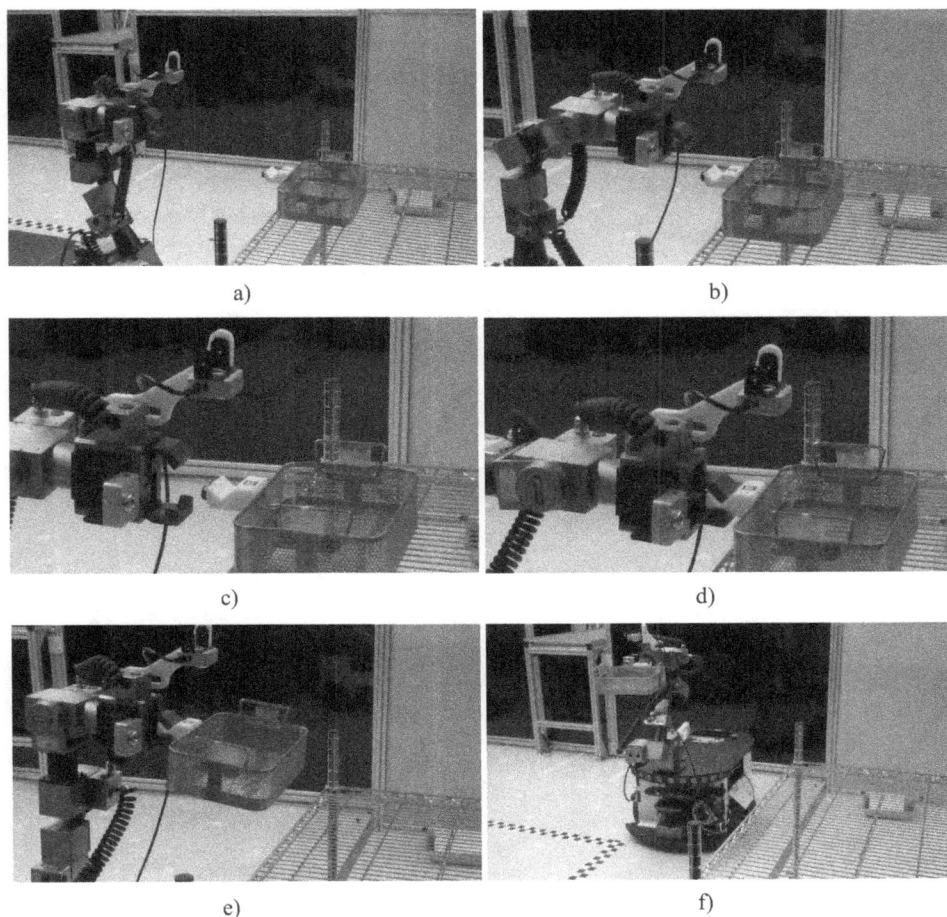

Fig. 3.8 Photo sequence of TrayBot performing manipulation during one of the experimental runs.

for the tray (b). TrayBot does not detect the tray after N line searches. Then, TrayBot moves forward to search the next N lines. During the search, TrayBot detects the tray. Then, motion trajectory is planned and carried out to reach the attachment on the tray (c). Then, TrayBot grasps the attachment by closing the two jaws (d), lifts the tray (e), and moves to the next position (f).

We placed the tray at 20 different locations in the working area on the cart surface and tested TrayBot's capability to pick up the tray. TrayBot successfully picked up the tray 100% of the time. Due to errors generated by camera distortion and/or the limitation of the joint angles, the grasp point computed by the robot can have errors =up to 1cm. Due to these errors, TrayBot could grasp the attachment on the tray but not very precisely. However, this is mitigated by our self-aligning

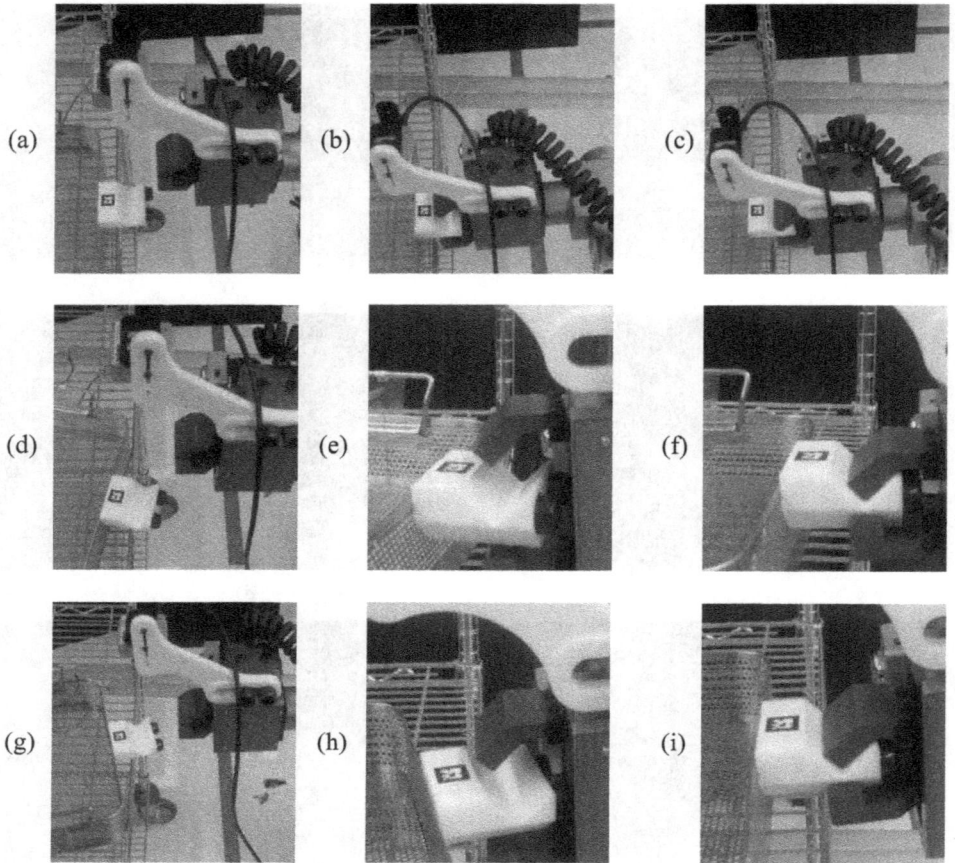

Fig. 3.9 Grasping the tray at three different orientation. Each row shows a sequence of grasping action at different angles: (a-c) $\theta = 0°$ (d-f) $\theta = -15°$ (g-i) $\theta = 15°$

gripper.

3.5.2 *Angle Tolerance of the Gripper*

As shown in Fig. 3.9, we place the tray with three different orientations with $\theta = 0°$, $\theta = -15°$, and $\theta = 15°$. In all three cases, TrayBot is able to successfully grasp the tray and it can use its custom gripper to align the orientation of the tray with the gripper.

We place the tray at four different locations and test the maximum tolerated angles as shown in Fig. 3.10. At each location, the orientation of the tray changed from $\theta = -30°$ to $\theta = 30°$. We then calculate the success rate of the grasping manipulation and the maximum angle that the robot can use its end effector to handle. This experiment is designed to test the *error tolerance* of using our cus-

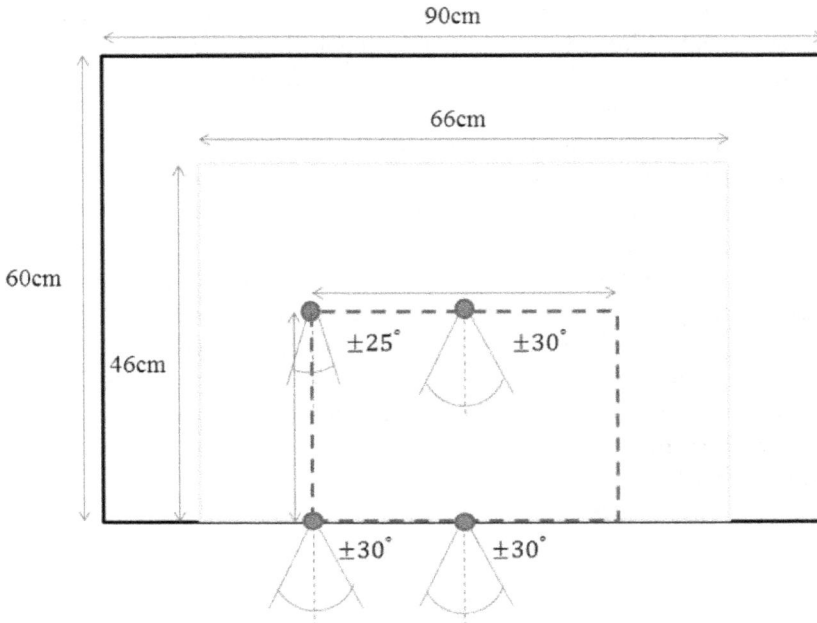

Fig. 3.10   Maximum tolerated error angle for different locations on the cart.

tomized gripper to grasp the attachment not the *orientation tolerance range*. For example, the tray can be placed on the cart with $\theta = 50°$, and the robot can change the orientation of its end effector to 50° to grasp the attachment. However, if the vision part is not precise, error exists for the angle computed by the fiducial marker detection algorithm. We want to test how much error our customized end effector can handle. In order to simplify the testing, we keep the orientation of the end effector at 0° and change the orientation of the tray.

When the tray is located at the top left spot, the maximum tolerated error angle is about ±25°. For the remaining three spots, the maximum tolerated error angle is ±30°. This is reasonable because the top left location is the farthest point the robot arm can reach. Different joints have different limitations on joint angles. Some joints may not reach the desired angles for desired manipulator configurations, but this will not affect the overall system performance. Based on these experimental results, we can conclude that our method of developing an integrated navigation and manipulation system could satisfy the requirements of our project.

3.6   Conclusion and Future Work

This chapter introduces our integrated navigation and manipulation system; named TrayBot, which can pick up trays from a cart, navigate within a sterile processing center, and place the trays on desired tables. Planning, decision-making, localization, navigation, and vision-based manipulator control are incorporated into this system. Special design of end effector contributes to the error handling capability. The experimental results demonstrates that our method is effective and can satisfy the requirements of our projects. TrayBot could easily be adapted to other projects which require navigation and manipulation for robotic transporting.

We want to further investigate a couple of issues in our future research. In our system, we are now using chilitags, which enables fast image processing and detection. However, in some cases, it is not reasonable to put additional fiducial markers on objects. We plan to analyze the features of the objects, e.g., shapes and textures to improve the performance of the vision detection module. Additionally, current decision making process in our system is deterministic. In the future, we would like to investigate integrating task-constraints and environment-constraints on different levels to increase the flexibility and robustness of the planning and decision making modules.

Chapter 4

Vision-based Instrument Singulation

In this chapter, We describe a novel single-view computer vision algorithm that identifies the next instrument to grip from a cluttered pile. This research was motivated by the challenges of perioperative process in hospitals today. Current process of instrument counting, sorting, and sterilization is highly labor intensive. Improperly sterilized instruments have resulted in many cases of infections. To address these challenges, an integrated robotic system for sorting instruments in a cluttered tray is designed and implemented. A digital camera is used to capture an image of a cluttered tray. A novel single-view vision algorithm is used to detect the instruments and determines the top instrument. Position and orientation of the top instrument is transferred to a robot. Experiments have demonstrated high success rate of both instrument recognition.

4.1 Introduction

The perioperative setting is considered the most resource intensive section of the hospital. Automating the process has the potential to significantly address current safety and efficiency concerns. A key component, which is also the goal of the computer vision algorithm described in their chapter, involves a robotic arm picking up individual instrument and sorting them into different bins or stacks.

Existing approaches to automating the sorting process are expensive and are limited in their capabilities. The state-of- the-art solution, RST's PenelopeCS is designed to automate several key functions for the clean side of the sterile supply [LaSelle (2011)].A human operator first separates the surgical instruments from a container and places them on a conveyor belt one at a time. Then a six-axis robotic arm fitted with a magnetic gripper picks up a single instrument from the belt. A machine vision system or a barcode scanner is used to identify instruments and sort them into stacks. This requires additional infrastructure as well as human operation at critical junctures; thus limited in an unstructured environment where surgical instruments are cluttered in the container.

There are several challenges in designing such an automation system. First, the surgical instruments often have very similar characteristics. This makes it difficult for vision-based algorithms to recognize them from an unordered pile. Second, instruments are made of shiny metal. Optical effects such as specularities and interreflections pose problems for many pose estimation algorithms, including multi-view stereo, 3D scanning, etc. Without six degrees-of-freedom (DOF) pose, standard parallel or vacuum grippers will have trouble executing robust grip. Our solution addresses all these challenges effectively.

Our approach to automated sorting has two key elements: first, a vision algorithm that robustly identifies the instruments in a clutter, infers the occlusion relationships among the instruments, and provides visual guidance for the robot manipulator; second, a compliant end effector design , which can execute precise instrument gripping in cluttered environment with only a 2D reference point as picking location (see Chapter 5 for details). This flexibility of the end effector is important because determining a weak 4-DOF pose in 2D space is easier and potentially faster than computing an accurate full 6-DOF pose due to the optically-challenging nature of the surgical instruments. To our knowledge this is the first instance of an automated sorting solution that is robust to handling a varied instrument suite.

The rest of the chapter is organized as follows. Section 4.2 outlines the related work. Section 4.3 discusses the details of our vision algorithm. The results are summarized in Section 4.4. Section 4.5 outlines a brief plan for future research.

4.2　Related Work

Picking individual items from an unordered pile in a container or in unstructured environments has been a popular research topic for several decades [Rahardja and Kosaka (1996)]. Some of the recent developments rely on active sensing. For example, Kinect sensor has been used to acquire a depth map of the scene [Papazov et al. (2012)][Nieuwenhuisen et al. (2013)]. Then, known 3D object models are matched to the acquired point clouds. Choi et al. use a structured-light 3D sensor to capture 3D models of objects in a box [Choi et al. (2012)]. A Hough-voting approach based on oriented surface points is used to estimate pose of the objects. A 3D laser scanner is used in PR2 for mobile manipulation in an unstructured environment [Chitta et al. (2012)]. These 3D sensors will have difficulty capturing specular objects such as surgical instruments.

Some previous work has aimed to provide a solution for bin-picking shiny objects in industrial settings. Shroff [Shroff et al. (2011)] propose a system that extracts high curvature regions on specular objects using a multi-ash camera. Multi-view triangulation on these features is then used to obtain the object pose. Rodrigues et al. [Rodrigues et al. (2012)] build an imaging system with a single camera and multiple light sources. A random fern classifier is trained to map the appearance of small patches into poses. Liu et al. [Liu et al. (2012)] use a multi-flash camera to obtain good depth edge information and use fast directional chamfer matching to match templates onto the input image for robotic bin-picking. Pretto et al. [Pretto et al. (2013)] use a single camera and a large diffuse light source mounted over the container. Their approach estimates a 6-DOF pose for planar objects based on a candidate selection and refinement scheme. In their experiments, each container only contains one object type. Both this method and the chamfer matching based methods rely on minimizing a cost function over a parameter space of transformations for each template. Computation time scales linearly with the number of templates. While for our approach, the computation time depends on the actual number of objects and their image-space intersections instead of number of templates. This makes our method suitable for handling large variety of surgical instruments. Large number of templates also increases the proportion of false correspondences for template matching, especially when the surgical instruments are very similar. Moreover, the matching cost is highly dependent on the shape and size of the objects and occlusions. Thus, it is problematic to simply pick the object with the smallest matching cost. In Fig. 4.1, we applied the Fast Directional Chamfer Matching algorithm by Liu et al. [Liu *et al.* (2012)] on one of our input images with five instruments. We searched for all five templates and highlighted the instrument with the smallest cost, which is not a good candidate for picking. Finally, our method uses one single DSLR camera without the need of multiple lights and multi-views. Thus, it is cheaper and easier to implement. Instead of 6-DOF pose,

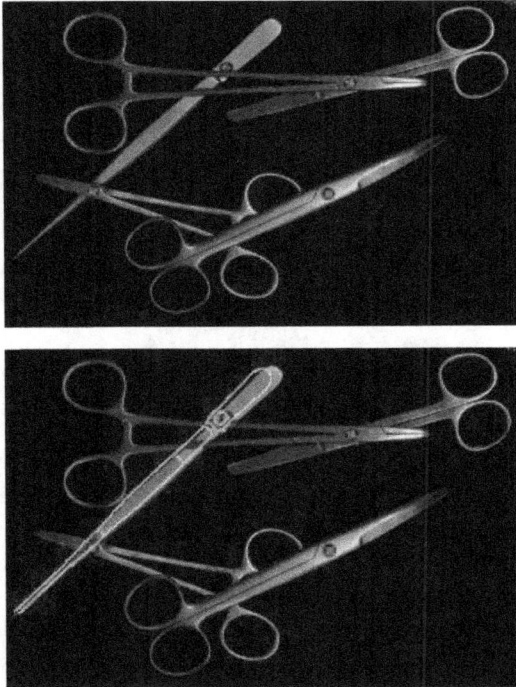

Fig. 4.1 Apply the Fast Directional Chamfer Matching algorithm [Liu *et al.* (2012)] on the surgical instrument data. (top) Input image. (bottom) The best match is highlighted.

weak 4-DOF pose in 2D space is estimated to guide the gripper.

Data-driven approaches are also popular among robotics researchers. Collet et al. [Collet *et al.* (2011)] develop a multi-view approach that can recognize all objects in the scene and estimate their full poses. Their approach relies on learned models for the objects using SIFT descriptor. Due to strong similarities among surgical instruments, such a data-driven method will be difficult to carry out.

Occlusion reasoning has also gained attention in the vision community. This problem can be solved by modeling local inconsistency for the occluders [Wang *et al.* (2009)]. However, for surgical instruments, occluders will have similar appearance as those being occluded. Alternative approaches focus on learning the structure of occlusions from data [Kwak *et al.* (2011)]. This method could potentially work for our application but requires a training stage. Hsiao and Hebert [Hsiao and Hebert (2012)] propose a multi-camera approach to model the interactions among 3D objects. Our approach compares the single input image with different hypotheses generated based on all possible occlusion configurations. We use a contrast invariant feature descriptor that is robust to the challenging optical effects.

4.3   Vision-based Surgical Instrument Singulation

Our vision system is designed for operation on both sides of the sterile processing. It first identifies the surgical instruments within the container for counting purpose. Then, it performs an occlusion reasoning step that determines what instruments are on top of the pile and not occluded by others. These instruments are candidates for gripping and singulation. Finally, a grip point is determined and communicated to the robot manipulator. The robot picks up the surgical instrument, and places it in an appropriate location in the target surgical kit. This process is repeated again until all objects are removed from the container. To achieve these goals, we use a high resolution DSLR camera that is mounted over the robot manipulator. The camera looks downward at a pre-defined region within the robot's work space.

4.3.1   *Surgical Instrument Identification*

In recent years, automated tracking of surgical instruments has been gaining popularity among healthcare organizations [Key Surgical (2018)] [Censitrac (2018)]. Individual instrument tracking beyond tray level improves infection control and provides a mechanism for process improvement and root cause analysis. Typically, each surgical instrument is equipped with a 2D data matrix barcode encoding a unique ID for the tool. These barcodes are small ranging from 1/8 to 1/4 inch in diameter, making them suitable for tracking objects with small flat surfaces such as surgical instruments.

Our system uses KeyDot® [Key Surgical (2018)] for instrument identification. A commercial off-the-shelf barcode reading module 2DTG [2D Technology Group (2018)] is used to locate and read the identifications of all the visible barcodes from

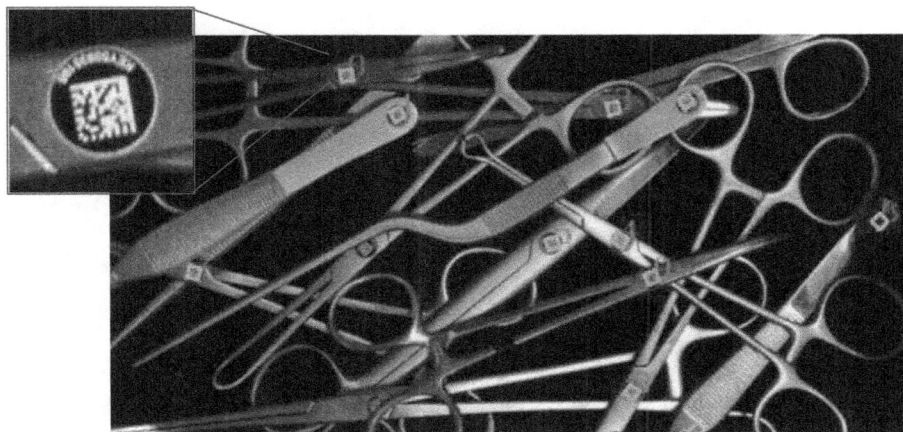

Fig. 4.2 Decoded barcodes are highlighted using small bounding boxes. There are a couple of missed detections due to occlusion. (Inset) Zoom-in view of one of the barcodes.

high-resolution images. To ensure identification, we place two barcodes on each side of an instrument. We assume flat objects, such as surgical instruments with only two possible stable placements in the container. For non-flat instrument (e.g., forceps), a cap is used to close the tips, reducing the potential for alternate stable orientations that could limit barcode visibility. On dirty side, barcode visibility might be affected by biological remaining. In such case, the instrument will be treated as an exception. On the clean side, the instruments are free of debris and biological material. Barcodes will not be contaminated. Fig. 4.2 shows an image of the instruments in a container and detected barcodes highlighted in green.

4.3.2 *Localization and Pose Estimation*

Given the instruments' IDs, our system estimates a 4-DOF pose (i.e., 2D location, orientation, and scale) for each instrument. We achieve this by matching template of each instrument to its pose in the input image of the container. A library is populated with templates in a pre-processing step. Each template is an image of an instrument captured with black background. We segment the template by thresholding and removing small connected components. The foreground segmentation is also stored in the library as an image mask.

For each detected barcode within the container, we retrieve its corresponding template from the library. The barcode reading module not only reads the ID represented by the data matrix, but also detects the four corner points of the matrix barcode. By using the four corners on both the input image and the template image, we compute an initial affine transformation that brings the template into alignment with the instrument in the input image.

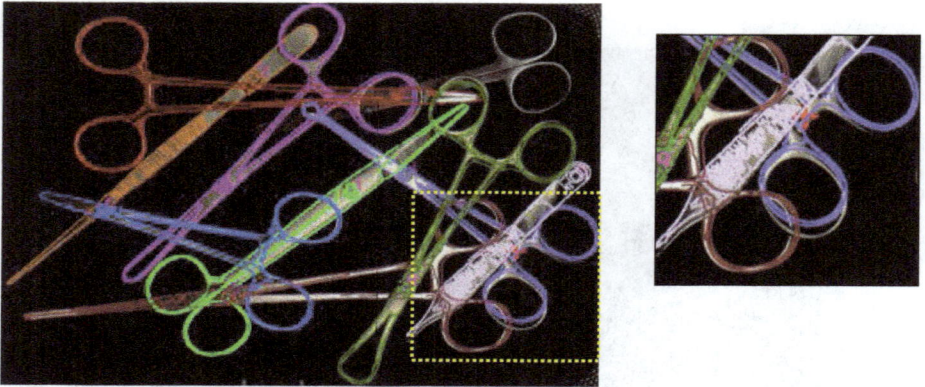

Fig. 4.3 Pose estimation using the four corners of the data matrices from both template and input image of the container.

Fig. 4.3 shows a visualization of the instrument localization and pose estimation step. We superimpose the edges of transformed templates onto the input image to show the effectiveness of the alignment step.

It is noteworthy that although projective transformation is more accurate for pose estimation of tilted surgical instruments, we use affine transform because it has fewer parameters (6 vs. 8), and because of the ability to obtain good initial guess from the data matrix corners. As we will discuss later, due to our robust occlusion reasoning algorithm and our compliant end- effector design, perfect pose estimation is not essential for the success of gripping.

4.3.3 *Occlusion Reasoning*

Given the poses of instruments whose barcodes are visible, our system then infers the occlusion relationship between each pair of intersecting instruments. This determines which instruments are not occluded by others and thus possible for the gripper to pick up next.

4.3.3.1 *Find the Intersections*

Our system first computes an occupancy map that models the intersections between all instruments. The occupancy map is a single channel image. Each bit of a pixel is assigned to one instrument. We first transform each template and its foreground binary mask using the computed affine transformation. We then store the transformed binary mask in the designated bit in the occupancy map. In this way, the intersecting region between two instruments can be easily determined by finding the occupancy map pixels that have the two corresponding bits. Fig. 4.4 shows an occupancy map and the intersection region between a few pairs of instruments.

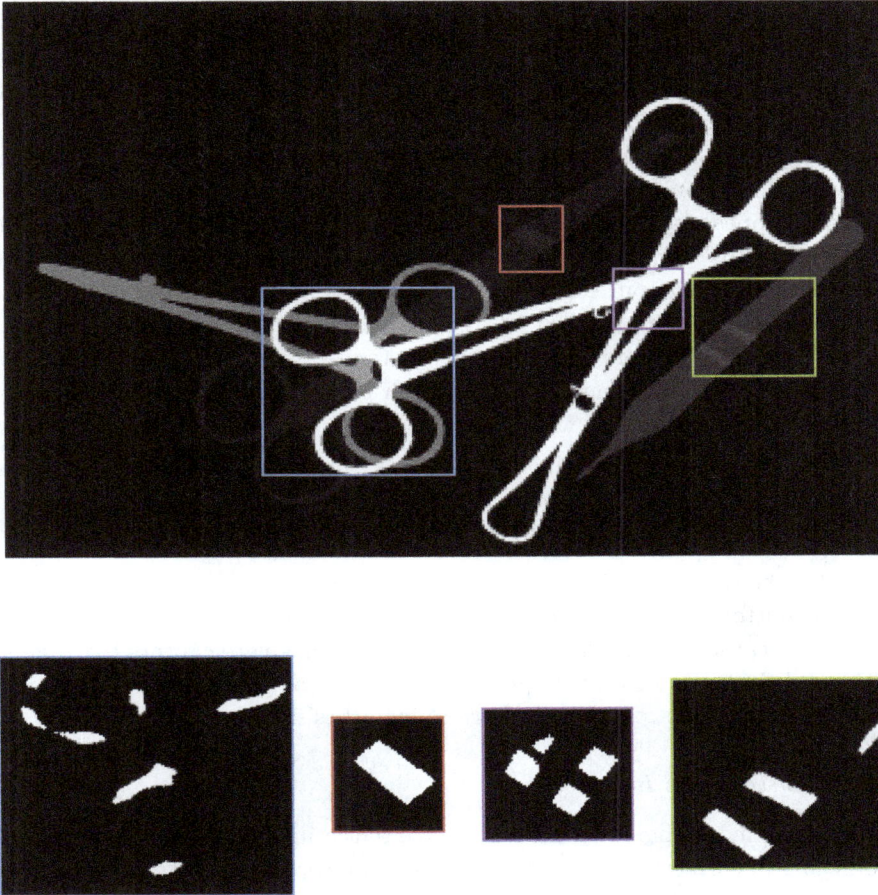

Fig. 4.4 (Top) An occupancy map of the instruments. Instruments that are assigned to a lower bit are expected to have lower intensity. (Bottom) Several dilated binary masks showing pair-wise intersection regions between instruments.

4.3.3.2 *Infer the Occlusions*

For every pair of intersecting surgical instruments A and B, there are only two hypothetical occlusion relationships: A occludes B or B occludes A. We synthesize two images, each of which corresponds to one of the two hypotheses (H_1 and H_2). The images are synthesized by transforming the templates to their poses in the input image and rendering them in two different sequential orders. The occlusion relationship can then be inferred by comparing the input image I against the two hypothesis images. Since H_1 and H_2 only differ at the intersecting regions and are identical for the rest of the pixels, we use the intersecting region computed from the occupancy map as a binary mask and only compare I against H_1 and H_2 within the masked region. We dilate the mask by a small amount to account for inaccuracy in the estimated instrument pose and to ensure all intersection regions are included in the binary mask.

To compare images, we use a descriptor called Edge Orientation Histograms (EOH) [Alefs *et al.* (2007)]. EOH descriptors are similar to the widely used Histograms of Orientated Gradients (HOG) [Dalal and Triggs (2005)]. EOHs are contrast invariant and only use edges instead of appearance information. They can handle large appearance changes due to varying lighting conditions, specularities, and interreflections among the surgical instruments. To reduce noise and focus on the more important contour edges, the input images are first blurred with a Gaussian kernel. We compute masked EOH (denoted as *meoh*) descriptors for image I, H_1, and H_2 and then compute Eculidian distances between the histograms. We use 2x2 overlapping blocks and 9 bins for each block, resulting in a 36 dimension descriptor. The hypothesis H with smaller histogram distance to the input image I is selected:

$$\hat{H} = \arg\min_{H_i} \|\text{meoh}(I) - \text{meoh}(H_i)\|_2, \text{where } i = 1, 2. \tag{4.1}$$

Fig. 4.5 shows a query image and two hypotheses. Notice that edges on the forceps (the bottom object) are different in the query image I and hypothesis images H_1 and H_2, because the templates and actual input image are captured at different lighting conditions. Due to strong presence of edges from the scissors (top object), our method is still able to select the correct hypothesis.

4.3.3.3 *N-Instruments Intersection*

In the case of more than two instruments intersecting at the same region, our method can still correctly predict the one that is on top of the pile. For example, if A occludes B and C, due to strong presence of A's edges in the query image I, the algorithm will predict A occludes B and C in two separate occlusion evaluations. The relationship between B and C is not important because we only look for the one instrument that is on top. Once A has been picked up, the relationship between B and C will be determined again in a later iteration. In other words, we are not trying to sort the entire set in one try. Because the pile of instruments may shift during each gripping, we need to capture an image and process the scene again before each grasping.

4.3.3.4 *Determine Picking Order*

We assume in most cases, there is no occlusion cycle among instruments (e.g., A occludes B, B occludes C, and C occludes A). This is a reasonable assumption considering all instruments are rigid, flat, and with tip closed. In case of instruments with occluded barcodes, because they will unlikely occlude the topmost instrument, our algorithm will still correctly predict the top one to pick.

a) Query Image *I*

b) Intersection Mask

c) H_1

d) H_2

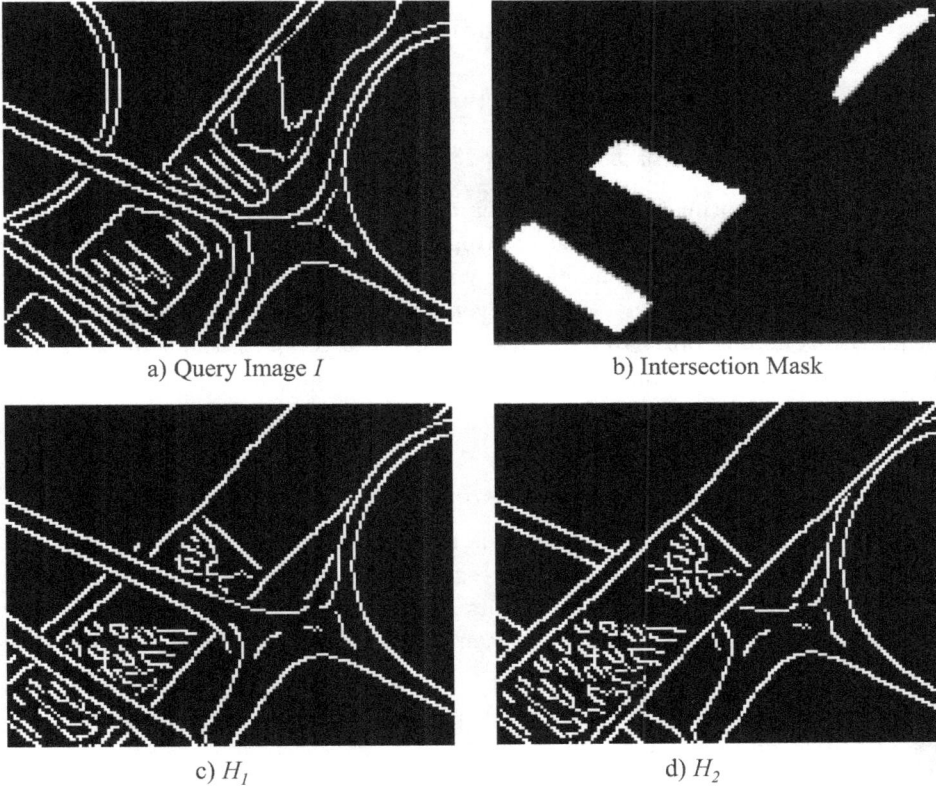

Fig. 4.5   a) A query image *I* generated by Canny edge detection on the input image and b) the associated intersection mask. c-d) The two synthesized hypotheses

Once all the occlusion relationships are determined, our algorithm finds the non-occluded ones. These can be instruments that do not intersect with others or that are on top of others. Our algorithm randomly selects one for the robot manipulator. The picking location for each surgical instrument can be determined empirically by a human operator in the template creation stage. Since our camera captures a top-down view of the instruments, the image plane is parallel to the robot's working surface. Thus, the picking location in the image space can be easily translated into the robot's coordinate system using a linear transformation. Because of our compliant end effector design, imperfection in this transformation does not affect gripping accuracy much. The picking height (normal to the image plane) is approximated based on known information for the given container and table surface heights.

Table 4.1   Results of Topmost Instrument Identification

Robot	# of Images	Correctly Identified Top One	Detect Rate
Baxter	229	213	93%
Adept®	192	182	94.7%

4.3.4   *Optimal Picking Location*

Alternatively, an optimal picking location can be determined for the target instrument. To do this, for every potential gripping point on the target instrument, we first define a surrounding bounding box, whose size is about the same as the diameter of the magnetic gripper. Then, we compute the area of the target instrument within the bounding box. We call this A_t. We also compute the sum of areas of all other instruments within the bounding box. We call this A_o. Then, for every possible point on the target instrument, we compute a ratio R:

$$R = A_t/A_o \qquad (4.2)$$

The point with the largest R value is the optimal picking location. By doing this, we maximize the contact area between the gripper and instrument; meanwhile minimize the chance of other instruments interfering with the gripping. The area of instrument within a bounding box can be efficiently computed by computing integral images on the occupancy maps.

4.4   Experiments

We implemented our surgical instrument singulation algorithm with a Nikon® D5200 camera and a PC with 3.2GHz CPU and 8G RAM. To detect small 2D barcodes on the instruments, we use images at 6000x4000 pixel resolution. In our experiments, we found that at least 70x70 pixels are required to decode a 2D data matrix barcode. For efficiency, our occlusion reasoning algorithm is performed at a much lower resolution at 1500x1000 pixels. To suppress small edges and noise, we use a 7x7 Gaussian kernel to blur images before computing histograms.

We performed 15 experimental runs each on Baxter and Adept® Viper arm using our vision based system. At the beginning of each run, the container is filled with approximately 12-15 surgical instruments. A total number of 421 images are captured and processed. The barcode detection on 6000x4000 images takes from 1.21 to 1.82 seconds depending on the number of barcodes in the view. The occlusion reasoning without pose optimization takes from 0.48 to 2.93 seconds to compute the gripping location depending on the complexity of the clutter.

Table. 4.1 shows quantitative results for our experiments on Baxter and Adept®. Our vision algorithm successfully detects the topmost instrument or the one that is least occluded for 93% of the time on Baxter and 95% on Adept®. The difference in success rate is due to the difference in tray size and camera height in two different configurations.

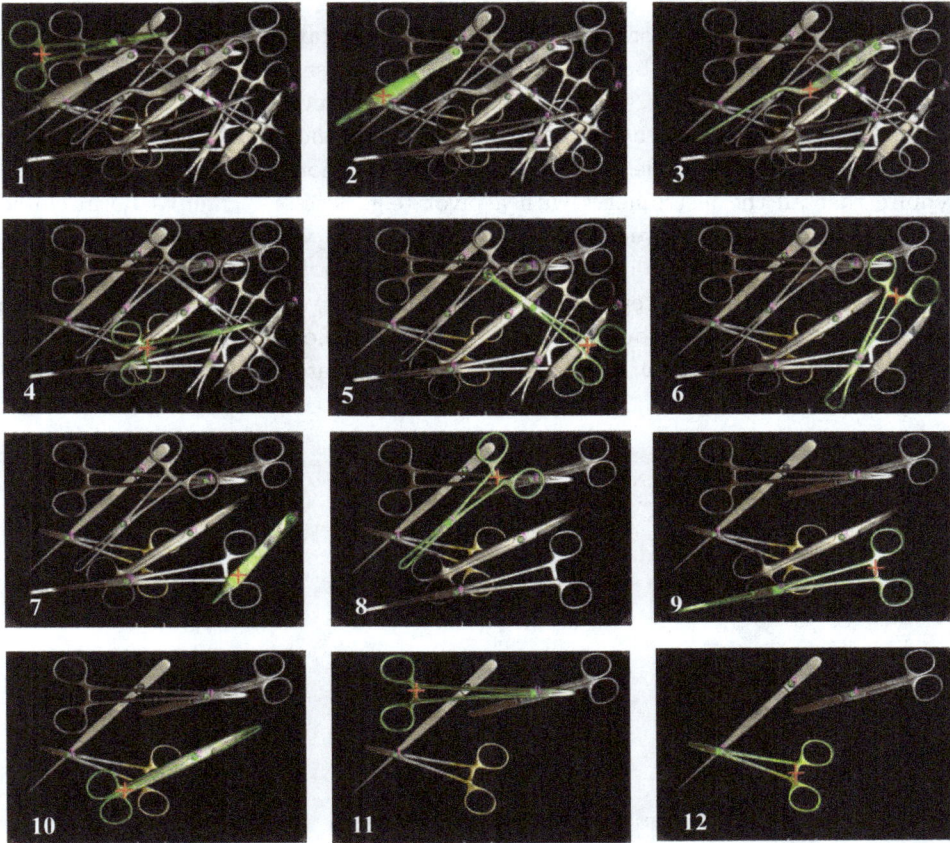

Fig. 4.6 Camera views from an experimental run of our robot manipulator. Each image shows the container before gripping. The target instrument is highlighted in green. The 2D reference point for gripping is marked by a red +. The final two images are omitted because there is no occlusion.

Fig. 4.6 shows the image sequence captured by the camera before each grip in one of the experimental runs using Adept®.

4.5 Conclusion and Discussion

We developed a vision algorithm for identifying the topmost surgical instruments from a container. Our vision algorithm is robust against optical challenges such as changing light conditions, specularities, and interreflections among the surgical instruments. The design of a compliant electromagnetic gripper (see next Chapter) enables us to only solve a 2D pose estimation problem instead of more challenging 3D pose. The algorithm can be extended to applications involving other mostly planar objects, such as certain industrial parts.

In the future, we will work on error handling. For example, a vision-based object verification algorithm can be used to determine whether the top object is occluded by some unknown objects. In the case where a wrong instrument is gripped, a verification step using an additional camera can be incorporated to verify if the singulated instrument is the one determined by the vision algorithm. Currently, we require that all the instruments with a pivot (e.g., scissors, clamps) be in closed position. In the future, we would like to extend the vision algorithm to handle opened instruments. This involves identifying the instruments, finding the pivot location, and performing template matching on the two portions separately. We would also like to extend our system for picking up non-planar objects. We can achieve this by placing a barcode and creating a template at each stable position of the object.

Chapter 5

Instrument Sorting Robots

In this chapter, we introduced two robotic systems that are capable of picking-up surgical instruments from a tray and placing the surgical instruments into different locations according to the instrument types. One of the robots is used on the dirty side of the sterile processing center and it is implemented using a RethinkRobotics® Baxter research robot. The other robot is used on the clean side of the processing and it is implemented using a clean room certified Adept® Viper arm. The pick-n-place manipulation is integrated with the vision component detailed in Chapter 4 and a special electromagnetic gripper. We tested our system in a lab-based environment and the system performance satisfies the requirements of the project.

5.1 Introduction

Typically, a sterile processing center has a dirty side and a clean side. On the dirty side, instruments are washed and disinfected manually. Debris and biological material are removed from the instruments. On the clean side, instruments are counted, built into surgical kits, and subsequently sterilized. The different operational conditions and accuracy requirements of the two sides justify different designs for each side.

When surgical instruments are returned from ORs, they are simply placed in a container without ordering. The job of the dirty side robot is to pick up the instruments and sort them into several empty containers based on instrument types (e.g., scissors, tweezers). This is to facilitate the manual cleaning process, because different types of instruments may require different handling procedures. For this purpose, we use a Baxter research robot. Baxter is a new type of robot that can work safely next to people due to its compliance design. This allows sterile processing nurses to perform essential tasks around the robot. The nurse first takes the dirty tray from the storage cart and puts all instruments onto a designated area on Baxter's working table. Then, Baxter separates the instruments into different trays. Then the nurse brings these trays to the sink and washes them manually. Finally, the nurse places the empty trays back onto Baxter's working table for the next round of instruments. Due to the lower accuracy of Baxter compared to typical industrial robots, picking error happens more often with Baxter. However, this is not a problem since the sterile processing nurse can manually correct these errors while washing the instruments.

After the decontamination step on the dirty side, the instruments are moved onto the clean side for further processing. The job of the clean side robot is to count the instruments, pick them up, and place them into pre-defined locations of a surgical kit. For this purpose, we use a clean room certified six-axis Adept® Viper S650 arm for its higher accuracy. We enhance both the Baxter robot and Adept® Viper arm with our vision system described in Chapter 4.

The rest of the chapter is organized as follows. Section 5.2 outlines the related work. Section 5.3 discusses our end effector design. Section 5.4 and Section 5.5 describes the dirty side robot and clean side robot respectively. The results are summarized in Section 5.6. Section 5.7 outlines a brief plan for future research.

5.2   Related Work

Pick-and-place robots are a mature class of robots that have increasingly become a critical functional component in the manufacturing and healthcare domains. Robotic solutions in these domain range from surgical robots to the low-cost Baxter® [Rethink Robotics (2018)] for close operations with humans. Despite the significant advances in the field, a key open technical challenge in the domain is the need for low-cost, adaptive end effectors that can be used for precision operations.

Commonly-used and commercially-available robot grippers include vacuum grippers, parallel grippers and magnetic grippers. Vacuum grippers are widely used in industry for its simplicity and gentle manipulation. However, they have difficulty in handling irregularly-shaped objects with uneven surfaces; thus inappropriate for surgical instruments. Parallel grippers have high precision and repeatability. Most of them are custom made and tailored to specific applications. Recent advances in dexterous manipulation have made it possible to grip a large variety of objects with just a single gripper design [Dollar and Howe (2010)]. However, handling surgical instruments in cluttered environments is still very challenging. Sophisticated vision guidance with full 6-DOF pose estimation is needed to ensure reliable grip. Collision detection and avoidance is also required.

Magnetic grippers can generate enormous gripping force in a very compact form factor and can grip objects with irregular shapes. Because most metallic surgical instruments that require sterilization are ferromagnetic [ISO (2016)], PenelopeCS has used a magnetic gripper for surgical instrument manipulation [LaSelle (2011)]. This gripper has an electromagnet mounted on a 1-DOF spring-loaded base to allow for firm contact between the electromagnet and the surgical instrument. Such a design works well for instruments with known surface orientation (i.e., single object lying on a flat surface). However, system utility will be limited when used with instruments in a pile since 6-DOF pose estimation is required for obtaining contact surface orientation. To address this issue, we designed an electromagnetic gripper

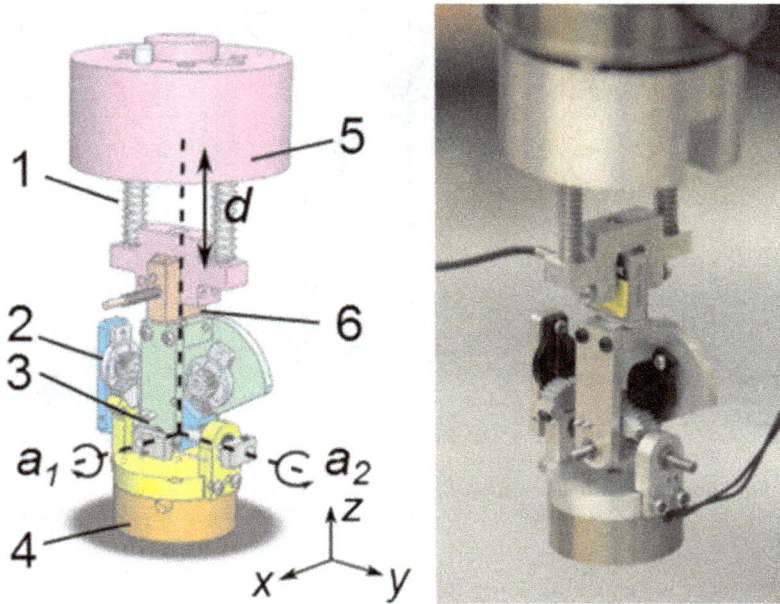

Fig. 5.1 Design and prototype of the electromagnetic gripper. 1: Spring for the z-axis compliance. 2: Rotary damper. 3: Torsion spring. 4: Electromagnet. 5: Adapter for Adept® Viper arm. 6: Load cell.

with 3-DOF compliance, which allows the electromagnet to passively reorient and conform to the instrument surface.

5.3 Our Compliant End Effector Design

The presented electromagnetic gripper is designed to grip a surgical instrument in a cluttered environment given a 2D reference point as the picking location. An annotated illustration and photo of the gripper is shown in Fig. 5.1.

The electromagnetic gripper has three passive joints: a prismatic joint along the z-axis and two revolute joints along the x and y axes. Each joint has a coil spring attached to the shaft; making these joints compliant. A rotary damper (ACE Controls® RTG2) is attached to each of the revolute joint shafts to prevent instrument oscillation after picking up and during transport. A load cell (Futek® LSB200, 5lbs) is used to measure the contact force between the electromagnet and the instrument. We use a threshold force F_t (e.g., $7N$) to determine when the electromagnet is in proper contact with an instrument (i.e., no gap between the electromagnet and instrument). An electromagnet (APW® EM137S) is attached at the bottom of the gripper. To reduce potential adherence between target instrument and adjacent instruments, the current of the electromagnet is modulated by a servomotor drive to generate a gripping force just enough to pick up the target instrument. We em-

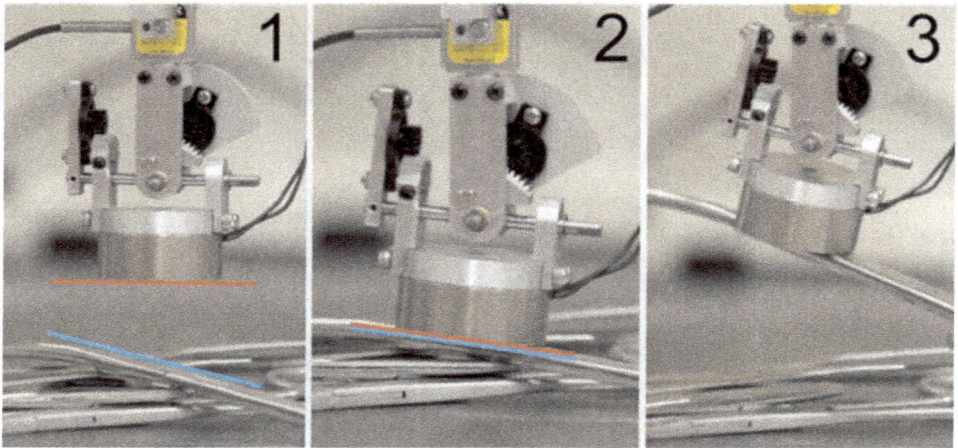

Fig. 5.2   Workflow of instrument gripping using our electromagnetic gripper. The red/blue lines approximate the surface orientation of electromagnet and instrument before and during contact.

pirically determine a picking force for each instrument and store them in a lookup table indexed by the instrument ID, which is provided by the vision system in real time.

An illustration of instrument pickup workflow is shown in Fig. 5.2. Given a 2D gripping location of a target instrument, a pick-up maneuver is completed with the following three steps:

(1) The robot arm moves the gripper to the gripping location and stops at a distance h above the instrument. Distance h is experimentally determined (e.g., *8cm*) to accommodate various pile height.
(2) The robot arm approaches the target along the z-axis. When the electromagnet comes in contact with the target, it re-orients itself to align with the instrument surface, regardless of their initial relative orientations. The robot controller constantly monitors the contact force until F_t is reached; indicating full contact with the target.
(3) The electromagnet is energized to pick up the instrument. The current is adjusted to the pre-calibrated value. The robot arm moves the electromagnetic gripper to lift the instrument and removes it from the tray.

One challenge with electromagnetic gripper is that the instrument may be slightly magnetized over time. Residual magnetism in surgical instrument must be removed to comply with surgical instrument requirement. Hence, the instruments after sorting must be demagnetized. Residual magnetism may also lead to instrument adherence to the electromagnet after setting magnet current to zero and cause an instrument drop failure during sorting. A solution for this issue is to oscillate the electromagnetic current I using the following equation,

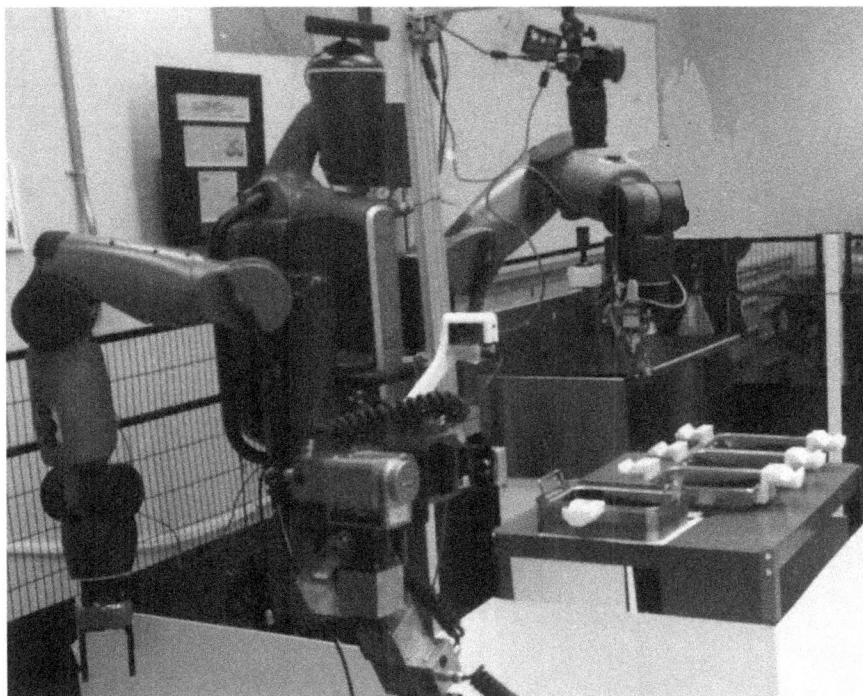

Fig. 5.3   A picture of Baxter sorting instruments on the dirty side of sterile processing.

$$I = I_0 e^{-t} cos(\omega t) \tag{5.1}$$

where I_0 s the electromagnet current for instrument picking. ω is manually chosen to be 20π for a balanced operation time and instrument-release success rate.

5.4   Dirty Side Sorter

There are a large amount of examples of deploying robots in manufacturing processes. However, how to place robots in the healthcare domain to perform certain tasks is still limited. In hospitals and healthcare centers, nurses and other workers are performing repeated work every day. Reducing their work load and protecting their safety at the same time is the goal of the current healthcare robotics research.

The difference between robotics research in manufacturing and healthcare are totally different. In most manufacturing situations, manipulated parts are determined and placed at certain locations for robots to pick and place. Pre-programed robots and pre-defined working environment could largely facilitate the automation. However, manipulation tasks for robots in healthcare domain are much more complex. Robots need to collect environmental information and make appropriate

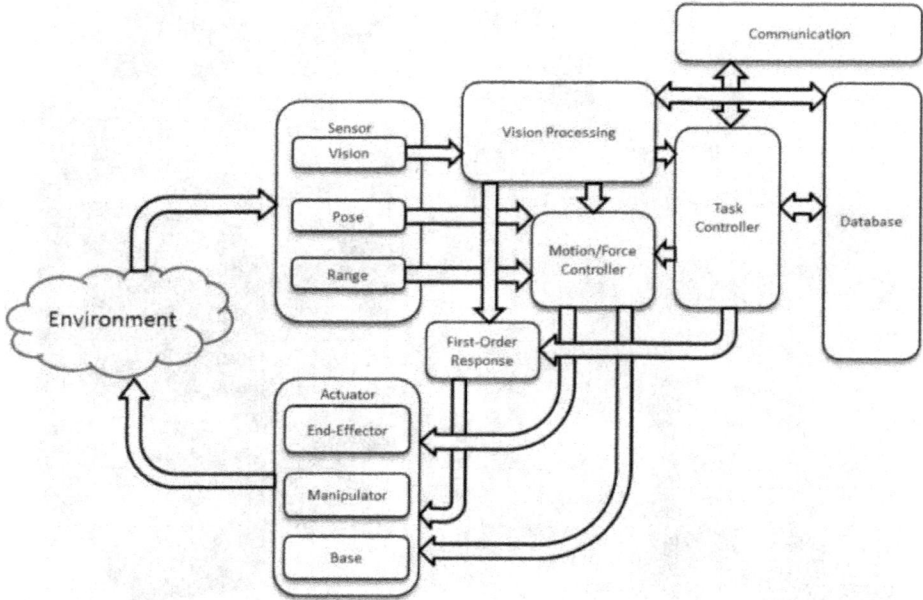

Fig. 5.4   Diagram showing the architecture of our dirty side sorting Baxter.

decisions to perform certain tasks. In order to achieve this goal, robots should be equipped with certain sensors to acquire environmental information, e.g., camera, infrared sensor, and laser sensor, etc.

In our system, we used Baxter research robot [Rethink Robotics (2018)] which is a new type of robots that can work safely next to people due to its compliance design as shown in Fig. 5.3. This allows sterile processing nurses perform essential tasks around the robot. Due to the lower accuracy of Baxter compared to typical industrial robots, picking error happens more often with Baxter. Thus, we use our special electrical magnet end effector (Section 5.3) to tolerate errors and imprecise detection in this system and increase the success rate of the overall system.

In this section, we highlight the architecture of the system and explain major components in this system in detail.

5.4.1   *System Architecture*

Fig. 5.4 displays the overall architecture of the system. Three control loops are developed at different system levels, including *Deliberative Task Control*, *Planned Motion Control*, and *Reactive Control*.

5.4.1.1 *Deliberative Task Controller*

This is the highest level control in this system, which receives information about the desired tasks from system manager, monitors the environment using vision processing component, and plans tasks for motion control layer.

5.4.1.2 *Motion Control*

Motion Control is responsible for planning the motion trajectories for all the tasks. The Baxter robot needs to move its end effector and its arm through all the via-points on planned motion trajectories. Closed-loop control algorithms are applied to ensure that the planned motion trajectories are followed.

5.4.1.3 *Reactive Control*

Reactive Control is used in our system to protect humans, the robot, and the environment, especially the surgical tools used. Whenever the robot detects any exceptions which are potentially dangerous to the robot and humans in the environment, a *First-Response* mechanism reacts immediately to stop the robot or modify the planned motions to avoid any possible damages to the overall system.

5.4.1.4 *Perception-Planning-Action*

From the perspective of functionality, this system is a typical *Perception-Planning-Action* system. Perception part includes the overhead camera for recognizing and locating the surgical tools, the encoders on the robot arm for kinematic and dynamic computing, and the force sensor on the end effector for grasping validation. Planning is related to scheduling and controlling, including higher level task planning, middle level motion planning, and lower level reactive planning, which deals with different goals at different levels.

5.4.2 *Major System Components*

In this sub-section, we discuss the major components in the system.

5.4.2.1 *Database*

The database is the memory component for the overall system, which stores required information for robots to use

Vision processing component requires pre-stored templates for surgical tools. In the database, all the templates are stored as images of the edges of the surgical tools. When a new surgical tool is added, this database will be updated accordingly.

Since we are using a task primitive-based planning system, the database also stores some basic task primitives: *Start, Stop, Pause, Vision Processing, Returning, Moving-Up, Moving-Down, Moving-Forward, Moving-Backward, Moving-Left,*

Moving-Right, Reaching, Grasping, and *Releasing.* These task primitives form the motion sequence.

5.4.2.2   *Task Controller*

The *Task Controller* sends out control signals to trigger different components directly and indirectly. There are two parts in this component: one is the task planning and scheduling, and the other is task monitoring and control, which are implemented in a *Finite State Machine (FSM)* and a *Decision Making Mechanism (DMM)* accordingly.

Triggered by the commands received from the *Communication* interface, the *Task Controller* generates a sequence of task primitives for Baxter to execute. The sorting task is a type of pick-and-place manipulation. A typical sequence of task primitives is generated as:

 (1) Vision Processing
 (2) Moving-Up
 (3) Moving-Right
 (4) Moving-Down
 (5) Reaching
 (6) Force Detection
 (7) Pausing
 (8) Grasping
 (9) Moving-Up
(10) Moving-Left
(11) Moving-Down
(12) Releasing

Due to the uncertainties within the system, the positions of the surgical tools are not fixed. Also, there may be some exceptions happening when the sorting is performed. Therefore, we implemented a simple DMM for the Baxter to make decision and handle different emergencies: there are several crucial rule-based decisions made by the robot by incorporating the sensory information and the current status of the performed task.

5.4.2.3   *Vision Processing*

We use the computer vision based instrument identification and sorting algorithm developed in Chapter 4 as the vision processing component for the dirty side sorting Baxter.

5.4.2.4   *Electromagnetic Gripper*

Baxter is originally designed with several finger type grippers, which have difficulty handling surgical instruments in a pile. We enhance the Baxter by equipping it with

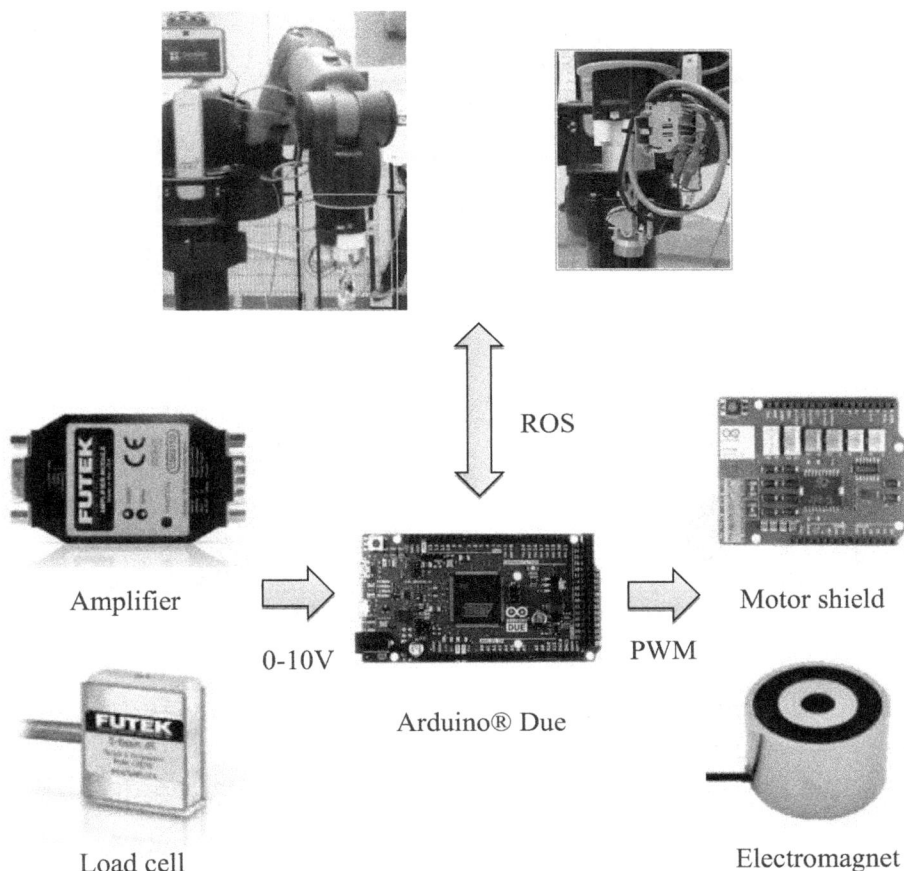

Fig. 5.5 Diagram showing that how the electromagnet gripper is integrated with with Baxter.

our custom designed electromagnetic gripper. To control the gripper, an Arduino®
Due microcontroller is used as a bridge between the gripper electronics and Robotic
Operating System (ROS) running on the Baxter. An Arduino® motor shield is
used to modulate the current in the electromagnet. The microcontroller reads force
sensor through an AD channel and sends a PWM signal to the motor shield. A
diagram of the electronic interface and a photo of the magnetic gripper mounted
on Baxter are shown in Fig. 5.5. Due to the fact that Baxter is compliant and
has up to 5mm of precision, the electromagnet tends to slide along the instrument
surface for less than a centimeter during contact. However, the electromagnet has
a diameter of 1.37 inches, less than 1cm position error may not be a significant
problem for instrument pick and place.

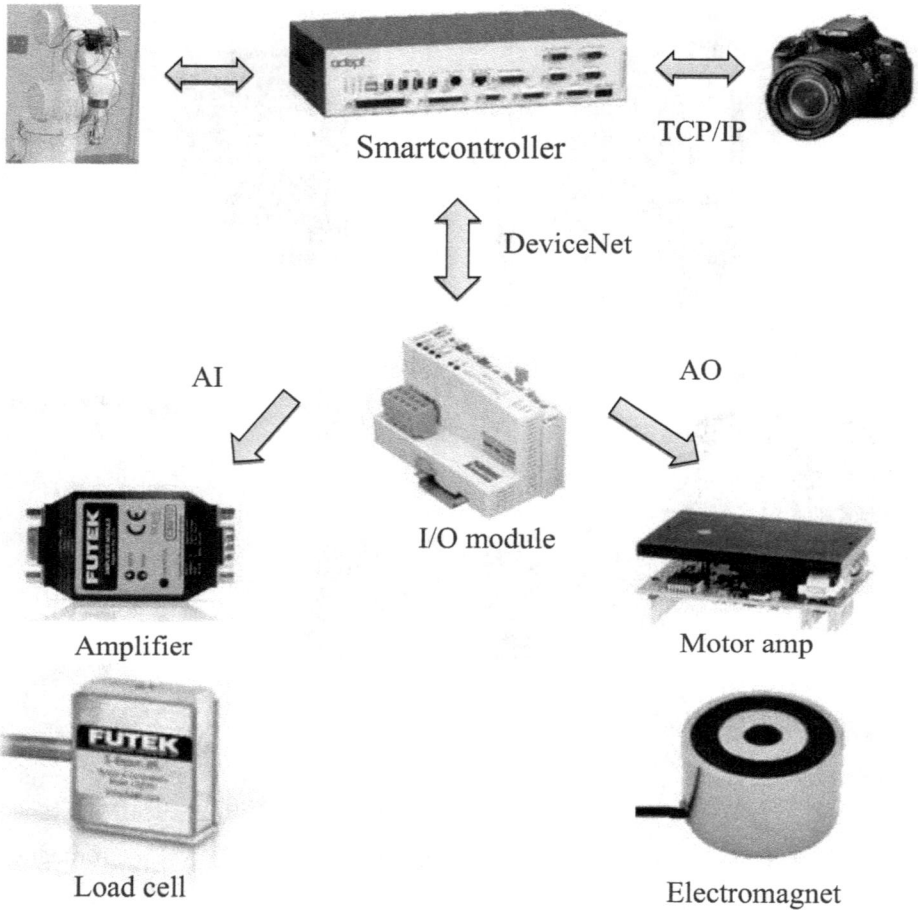

Fig. 5.6   Diagram showing the integration of the gripper with Adept® Viper arm.

5.4.2.5   *First-Order Response*

First-Order Response is a module making a decision significantly quickly to avoid any damage to the robot, the environment, and the devices. Although Baxter is a compliant robot which is safe to people, we still implement a software-based action component to provide more safety protection. In the sorting system, the biggest concern is that the robot hits the table with its gripper. This may harm the functionality of the gripper and will cause other issues in the sorting task. Therefore, the *First-Order Response* triggers a *Moving-Up* motion to avoid any further damage when the force detected on the gripper is larger than a threshold value. This simple fast motion generation method could largely reduce the chance of damaging the gripper and the robot.

5.5 Clean Side Kit-Builder

The Adept® Viper S650 robot arm and the electromagnetic gripper are controlled by an Adept® Smartcontroller. The load cell and the servomotor drive are interfaced with the robot controller through a Wago® DeviceNet analog I/O module. Figure 5.6 shows a diagram of the integration. Due to the lack of ROS on the Adept® Smartcontroller, the communication between the robotic vision system and the arm is via TCP/IP messages.

The Viper arm places the instruments into pre-defined slots in a surgical kit. We achieve this by first rotating the instrument to predefined orientation (e.g., upright) and then translating the instrument in the horizontal plane to bring the instrument into a target location in the kit.

5.6 Experiments

Tab. 5.1 shows quantitative results for our experiments on Baxter and Viper arm. When the candidate instrument is correctly identified, the success rate for singulation is 98% using Viper arm and 92% using Baxter.

Table 5.1   Results of Topmost Instrument Singulation

Robot	Correctly Identified Top One	Successfully Gripped	Success Rate
Baxter	213	195	91.5%
Adept® Viper	182	178	97.8%

5.6.1 *Experiments on Dirty Side*

The goal on the dirty side is for the Baxter to sort all the surgical instruments into different trays, which can be further processed by sterile processing nurses. To achieve this goal, three empty trays are placed on a table in front of the Baxter at the beginning of the task. Fig. 5.7 displays a typical manipulation process in this sorting task. In Fig. 5.7, the Baxter starts from the home position (1), moves to the cluttered surgical tools area (2), reaches a selected tool (3), uses its electrical magnet gripper to pick it up (4), moves to the position above the corresponding tray, and places the picked instrument in the tray (5).

Since Baxter is a compliant robot, and even when the vision algorithm successfully identifies, locates, and finds the gripping point on a surgical tool, sometimes robot may still pick up a different tool, or missed a tool. In our testing, the average success rate is 80%, and the variation depends on the configuration of the tools in the tray.

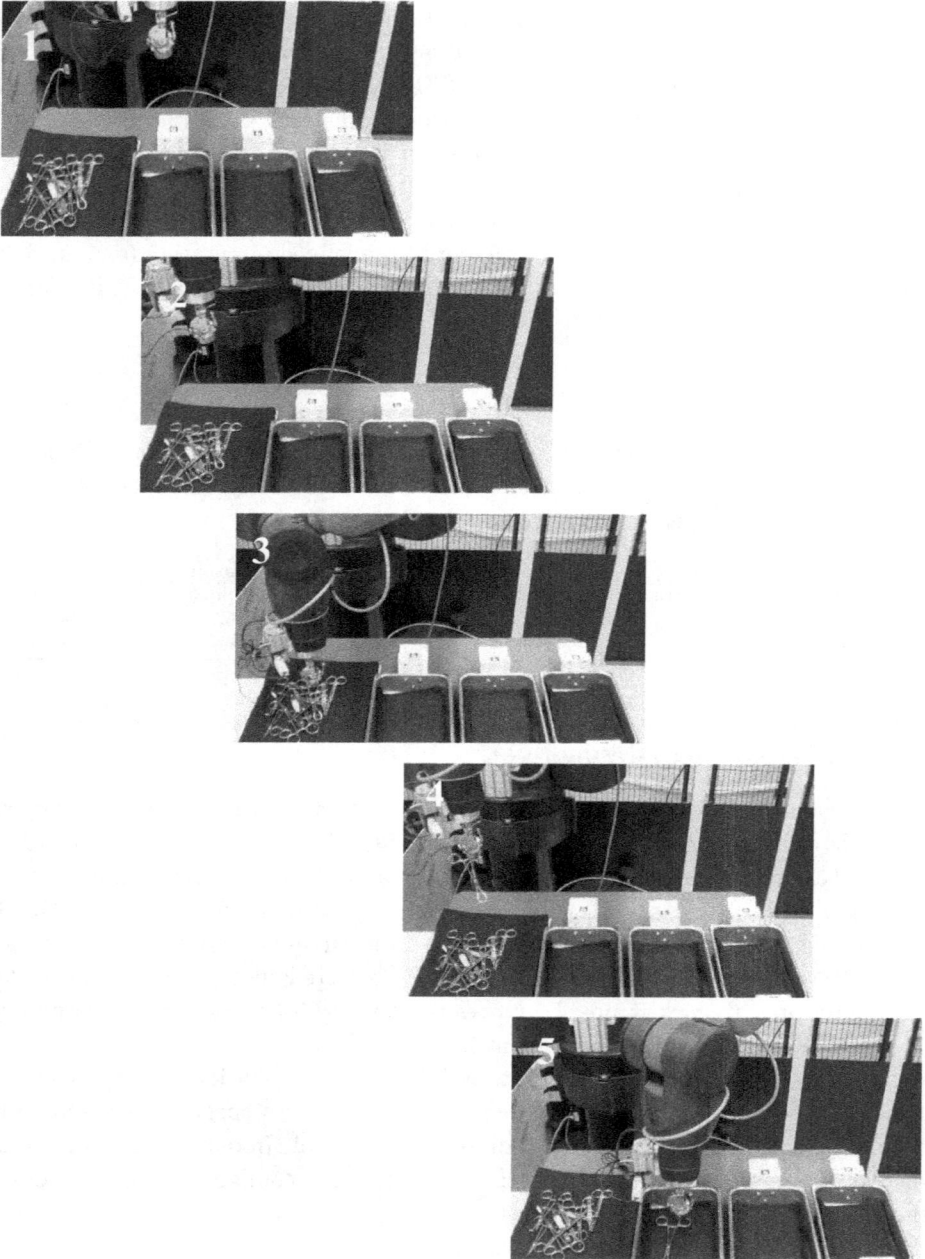

Fig. 5.7   Image sequence showing a typical manipulation sequence of Baxter sorting dirty instruments.

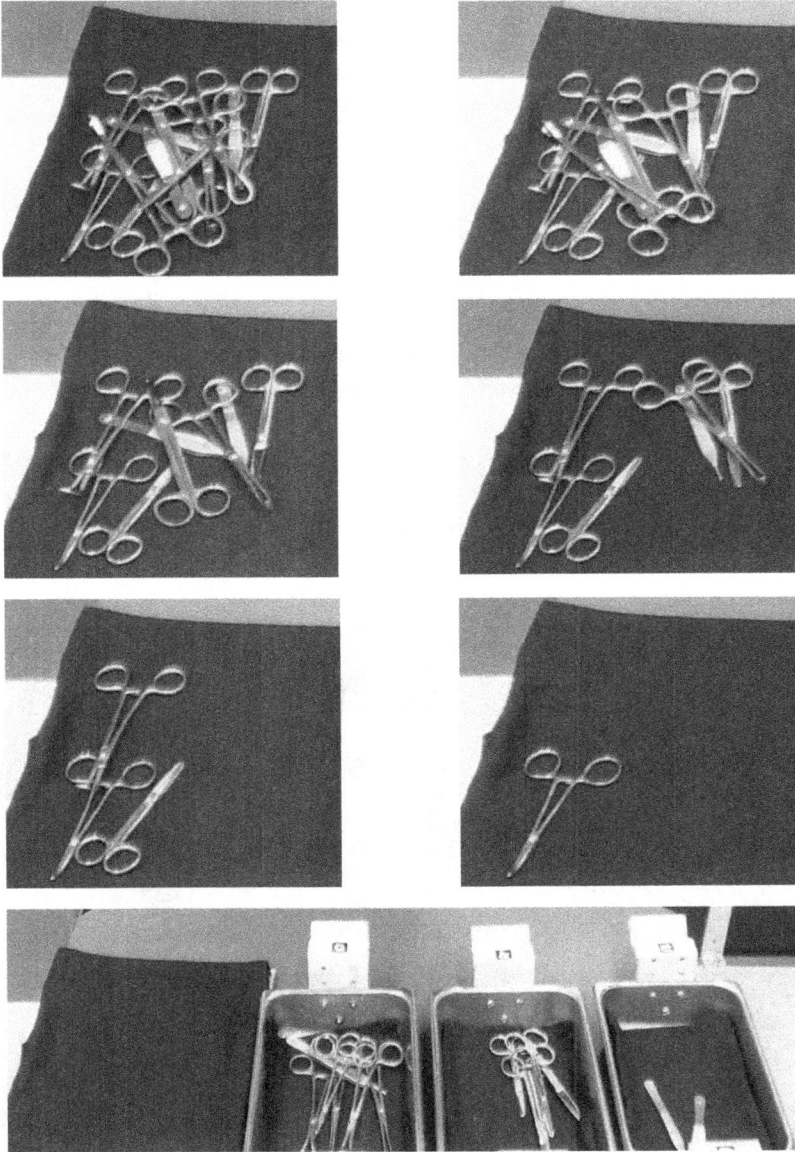

Fig. 5.8   Images showing a sorting process.

Fig. 5.8 displays a typical process of the sorting procedure. There are 12 tools that need to be sorted at the beginning of the process. Baxter successfully sorted 11 tools. However, one tweezer is misplaced into the left tray. This is because Baxter was supposed to pick up a clamp, but it picked up the tweezer instead due to the sliding caused by the compliance of the gripper. However, this is not a serious issue because after Baxter sorts all the dirty surgical instruments into trays, the trays will be washed manually at the ultrasonic cleaning station. At that time, the error can be corrected by the sterile processing nurse.

5.6.2   *Experiments on Clean Side*

In previous Chapter 4, we have shown a sequence of images where Adept® arm successfully singulated all instruments from a tray.

Occasionally, the robot manipulator fails to grip a target instrument. In Fig. 5.9 a), instruments A and B are aligned closely. The electromagnetic gripper makes contact with scissors B first and is not able to lift it up due to insufficient gripping force. The system decides to singulate the next available instrument after two failed tries. However, because instruments shifted during the failed attempt, there exists an occlusion cycle now in the scene (Figure 11b, D occludes C, C occludes B, and B occludes D). Since instrument D is least occluded, the system determines to singulate D. After removing D, instruments C and B shifted and are removed subsequently (Figure 11c-d).

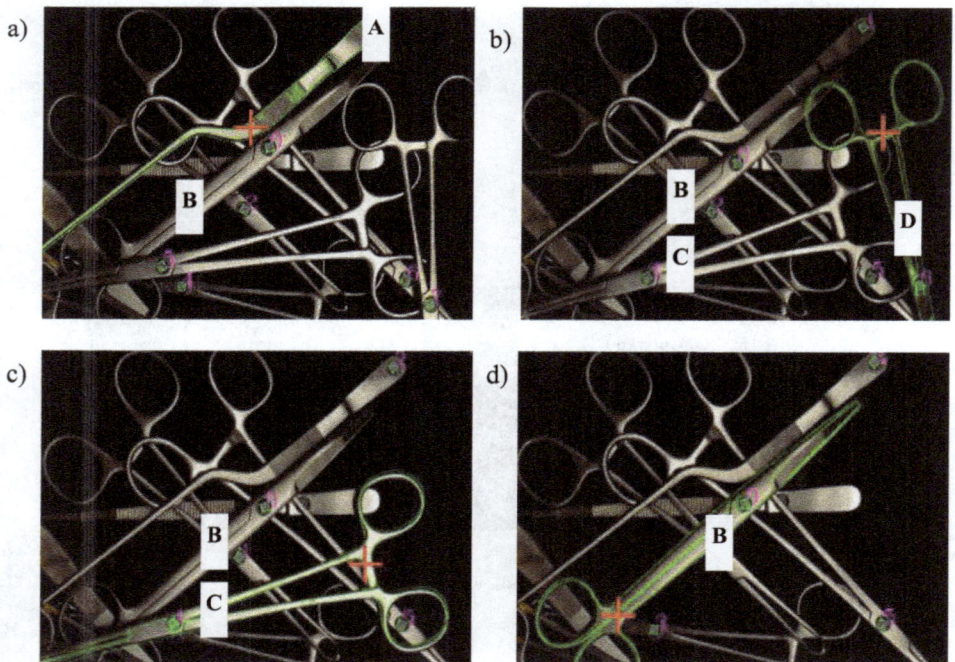

Fig. 5.9   Recovery from a failed attempt. a) Failed attempt when trying to remove instrument A. b) Instrument D is determined to be occluded the least. c-d) C and B shifted and are removed subsequently.

When the vision algorithm predicts an incorrect instrument that is still occluded (10 out of 192 images), the gripper either grips a wrong instrument or fails to grip due to insufficient force. For example in Fig. 5.10 a), instrument A is occluded by instrument B, whose barcode is not visible. The vision system is not aware of instrument B's presence and determines A is on top of the pile. The system attempts to grip instrument A but fails, resulting in shifted instruments in the container (Fig. 5.10 b). Instrument Bs barcode is now revealed. The robot manipulator is able to recover from the previous failure and successfully singulate instrument B.

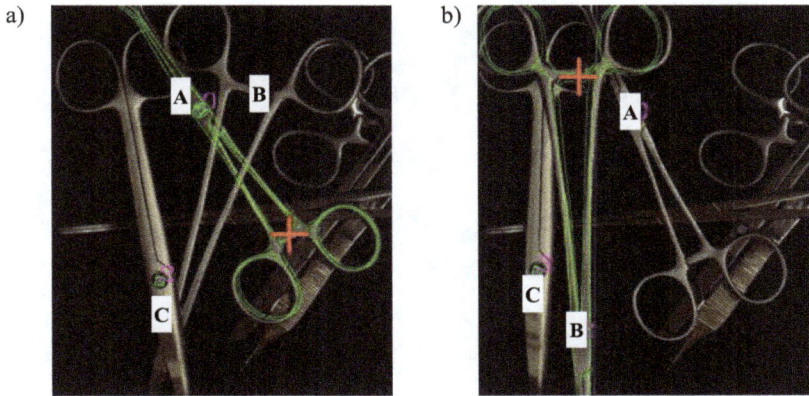

Fig. 5.10   A case where barcode is occluded. a) Vision system determines instrument A to be on top incorrectly. b) After a failed attempt, instruments shifted; resulting in a new configuration where the vision system successfully finds the topmost instrument B.

5.7   Conclusions and Discussions

In this chapter, we propose an integrated system design for robot to perform instrument sorting tasks on both the clean side and the dirty side of the sterile processing center. We explain the architecture design and specific component development in our system. Practical experiments are carried out on a humanoid robot RethinkRobotics® Baxter robot and on a clean room certified Adept® Viper arm to validate our design. The experimental results are satisfying and the robot can successfully perform the desired tasks.

In the future, we plan to improve the robustness of using the electrical magnet gripper on the compliant mechanism of the Baxter robot. This could reduce the misplacement rate and increase the overall system performance. One potential disadvantage with using electromagnetic gripper is the tendency for the instruments to be magnetized over time. However, this can be addressed with the use of a standard demagnetizer (e.g., Neutrolator®).

Chapter 6

Safe Robot-Human Collaboration

In this chapter, we discuss a vision-based cognitive system for robots to work in human-existing environment and keep the safety of the sterile processing nurses. An integrated system is implemented with perception, recognition, reasoning, decision-making, and action.

6.1 Introduction

Our automated robotic system involves several robots for both manipulation of surgical instruments and transportation of trays containing instruments. It is desired to deploy robots in such working environments to automate the process of transportation and sterilization and keep doctors and nurses from daily repetitive and harmful process. However, safety issues arise in situations where autonomous robots must work alongside humans. On the dirty side of the sterile processing center, we use a Baxter robot for sorting the dirty instruments and use a mobile TrayBot to transport trays around; thus, how to allow the robots to work alongside sterile processing nurses is a problem that needs to be addressed.

Safety in human-robot collaboration and human-robot co-existing environment is of highest priority. Safety concepts are defined following the famous Three Laws of Robotics [Asimov (2004)]:

- A robot may not injure a human being or, through inaction, allow a human being to come to harm.
- A robot must obey the orders given to it by human beings, except where such orders would conflict with the First Law.
- A robot must protect its own existence as long as such protection does not conflict with the First or Second Law.

From these laws, it is expected and required that robots, which work in human-existing environment, operate safely and provide signals related to safety issues to humans. From the social science prospective, safety rules should be enforced to enable robots to make suitable and correct decisions when they have to deal with complex task-relevant situations. From the engineering perspective, balance between productivity and safety should be well-maintained to achieve desired system performance. Under no circumstances, robots should sacrifice safety requirements to achieve unsafe productivity. Mathematically, this is a typical constrained optimization model of hierarchical description with different levels of priorities. The setting of these priorities is based on the Three Laws of Robotics.

However, different technologies incorporated into a safety system could affect the overall system performance. For example, different processing time impacts the synchronization between system components, especially in a distributed system design. Thus, integrated planning and coordination should be taken into consideration to achieve goals and objectives on all the layers and sub-groups of the overall system.

In this chapter, we propose a vision-based cognitive system for robots to work in human-existing environment and keep the safety of humans. An integrated system is implemented with perception, recognition, reasoning, decision-making, and action. Without using any traditional safety cages, a vision-based detection system is implemented for robots to monitor the environment and to detect the presence of human operators. Subsequently, reasoning and decision making enables robots to evaluate the current safety-related situation for humans and provide corresponding safety signals. The decision is made based on maximizing the productivity of the robot in the manipulation process meanwhile keeping the safety of humans in the environment.

The rest of this chapter is organized as follows: Section 6.2 discusses related work; Section 6.3 explains the system design; Section 6.4 evaluates the system using experimental results; and Section 6.5 summaries this chapter and proposes future work.

6.2   Related Work

For robots to work safely in human-existing environment, a traditional method is to put safety fence or cages around the robots. Some international standards enforce strict requirements on safety [ISO (2014)] [Fryman and Matthias (2012)]. However, this type of solution could significantly limit the mobility and ability of mobile robots. Moreover, when humans have to interact with robots and thus work inside the "cage", the traditional method cannot address the safety problem.

Some researchers developed innovative mechanisms to provide safety functions. Parmiggiani et al.   proposed a novel design for the joints of the iCub robot [Parmiggiani *et al.* (2014)]. These joints provide an overload protection mechanism that acts as a "passive" torque saturators. Hayashibe et al. addressed the safety problem of laparoscopic surgery by computing the robot position and organ shape via laser scanning [Hayashibe *et al.* (2006)]. Bast et al. used a stand-alone safety system to supervise the robot during the intervention of computer-assisted craniotomy [Bast *et al.* (2006)]. However, when integrating off-the-shelf robotic components, such safety system are not applicable.

There is growing interest in developing collaborative robots such as Baxter robot from the RethinkRobotics® [Guizzo and Ackerman (2012)] and UR series robots from Universal Robots company [Universal Robotics (2018)]. These types of robots aim to adjust manipulator motions to adapt to external forces, especially the interactive forces between robots and humans [Haddadin *et al.* (2009)] [Saito and Ikeda (2007)]. Collaborative robotics is promising, however, there is no collaborative mobile robot platform that satisfies our need for transporting surgical trays around the dirty side.

In our system, two robots are used on the dirty side of the sterile processing center where robots and sterile processing nurses collaborate together. One humanoid robot, Baxter robot, is equipped with a Kinect Sensor [Zhang (2012)] and is responsible for performing routine work and monitoring the overall environment especially the location of nurses and mobile robots. The mobile TrayBot moves around in the environment without actively searching for any human activities in the environment. The Baxter robot is able to gather environmental information and make decisions to generate corresponding actions. Although it cannot control the mobile robot directly, the Baxter robot is able to send out warning signals to human operators.

6.3 Methodology

We developed an integrated system to enable one robot to monitor the entire working environment using a Microsoft® Kinect sensor. The robot also makes decisions based on pre-defined criteria and sends out corresponding signals. Although safety modules are placed on robots to ensure human safety in the environment, there is a compelling need to augment the system's safety in cases where a human actively creates an unsafe operating situation, e.g., walking towards a robot or blocking a robot. Moreover, sometimes there are several humans in the environment. In order to achieve this goal, we must consider the integration of the perception, recognition, reasoning, decision-making, and action issues at the same time as shown in Fig. 6.1.

The overall system architecture is divided into five major components: *Perception, Recognition, Reasoning and Decision Making*, and *Action*. *Perception* module gathers information from the environment using a Kinect sensor, and from the robot using Encoders and Force Feedback Sensors. Based on the collected sensory information, our *Recognition* module is able to recognize the current activity of a detected human. Then, the *Reasoning and Decision Making* module makes a decision to select actions based on the current robotic, human and environmental information. Task selection is based on balancing the productivity of the manipulation task while satisfying the safety requirements. Finally, the *Actions* are carried out by the robot. We will discusses these modules in details.

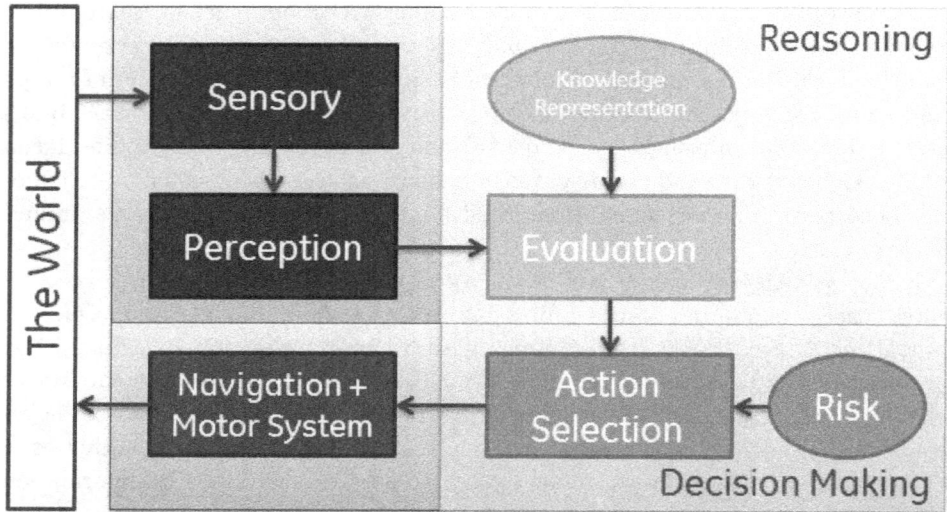

Fig. 6.1   A diagram showing our safety system architecture.

6.3.1 *Perception*

Perceptual information is used for Sensory-Motor Coordination and higher level processing. Perception includes not only obtaining the images, audio, and other sensory data from the environment, but also extracting useful information from them.

In our system, two types of sensors are used for Perception: Kinect sensor mounted on the head of Baxter for tracking human activities in the environment; encoder and force feedback sensors on the joints of robot arms and grippers for obtaining information from the robot.

The Kinect sensor powered with Kinect SDK can track up to six people in the environment in real time. After initialization, the Kinect sensor runs in a continuous loop of tracking the positions and poses of humans. The tracking results are organized in ROS message format and published on ROS topics for the recognition and reasoning modules to use.

6.3.2 *Recognition*

Human activities in the working environment are task-related; thus it is possible to predict human activities based on the current status of human and environmental information. In our system, we are more interested in the position of human bodies in the environment. Thus, we choose position of humans as the main observation feature used by the recognition model.

As shown in Fig. 6.2, in our system, the working environment of the dirty side of

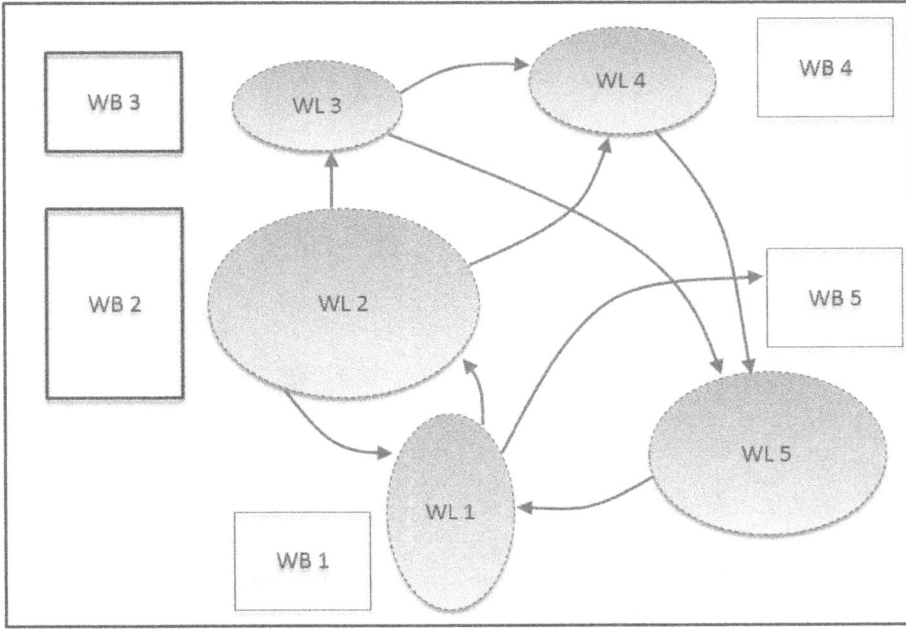

Fig. 6.2 Working environment represented as Work Benches(WBs) and Working Locations(WLs) of human operators.

the sterile processing center is described by five work-benches (WB) and five working locations (WL) for sterile processing nurses. Each working location is related to a corresponding state in the observation model. The transition probabilities between states are represented as:

$$a_{ij} = P(q_{t+1} = S_j | q_t = S_i), 1 \leqslant i, j \leqslant N \qquad (6.1)$$

The transitions are determined according to the pre-defined operation procedure of the dirty side sterile processing.

For each state, the Baxter robot uses the Kinect sensor to determine the locations of the nurses. However, because of the measurement errors of the devices, the environment errors, or even the errors of the nurses, the measured information is considered probabilistic. Then, the observation probability is defined as the probability of measured value v_k at time t while the current state is S_i:

$$b_{ik} = P(v_k | q_t = S_j), 1 \leqslant i \leqslant N, 1 \leqslant k \leqslant M \qquad (6.2)$$

Using the observation result, we can obtain the belief of which state the human is in, which follows a Gaussian distribution. The state with highest probability will be chosen and sent to *Reasoning and Decision Making* module for further processing.

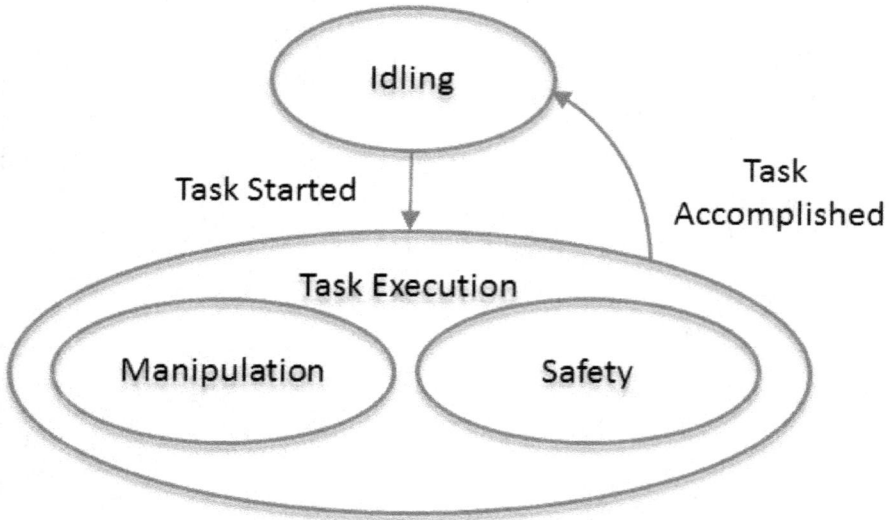

Fig. 6.3   Overall work flow of task execution.

6.3.3   *Reasoning and Decision-Making*

Two tasks are running simultaneously on the Baxter: *Manipulation* and *Safety*. This multi-task execution architecture highlights the importance of safety to provide a safe environment for humans and robots in the sterile processing centers. The *Reasoning* module receives the messages from the *Recognition* module. Using the environmental information and *a prior* knowledge, the *Decision-Making* module can make decisions and select actions based on the current task-relevant situation.

Fig. 6.3 displays the overall work flow of task execution. An important goal in *Decision Making* is to maximize the productivity while keeping the humans safe. When humans are not in dangerous areas, normal routine work shall not be interrupted. Otherwise, a naive solution would simply stop working every time the presence of human operators are detected.

Fig. 6.4 displays a state transition machine for the Manipulation task. In each operation, the Baxter reaches for the tool to be manipulated, uses a gripper to pick it up, and drops it in a desired tray. Fig. 6.5 shows the safety task implemented in our system.

Depending on the recognition results by using Kinect sensor, the Baxter robot recognizes the current locations of the human operators and predicts the future locations of the humans after a pre-defined time window. Based on the recognized and predicted results, the Baxter robot may quickly make a decision to switch states in the safety task. If a human is detected and he/she is far away from the TrayBot in the environment, Baxter keeps an eye on the human; if the human operator's proximity to the TrayBot is becoming a concern, Baxter sends out alarm signals; if

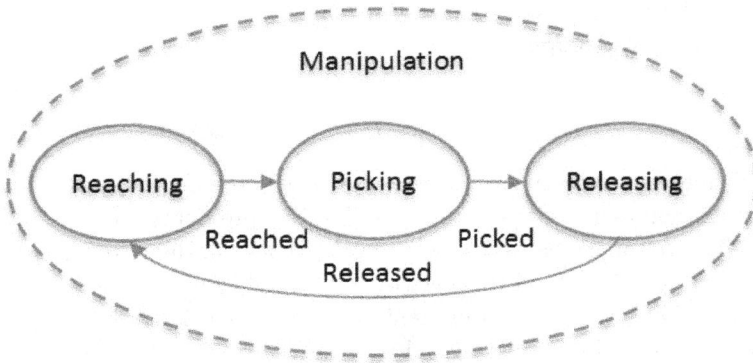

Fig. 6.4 State transition of the Baxter's Manipulation task.

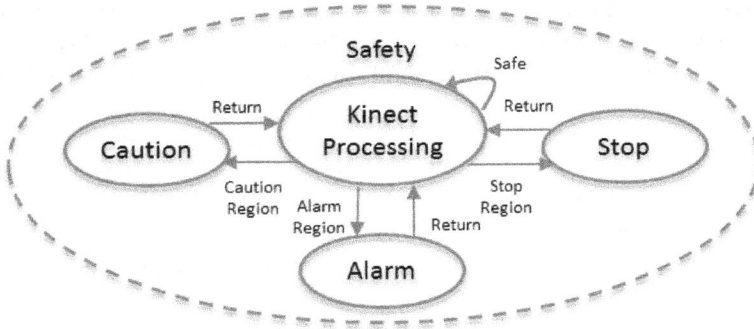

Fig. 6.5 State transition of the Baxter's Safety task.

Baxter predicts that the human is moving too close to a the TrayBot, and a collision is inevitable unless either the TrayBot or the human stops their current activity, it sends a STOP signal to the system operator.

6.3.3.1 *Maximize Productivity*

In our system, productivity refers to normal operations in the process without any interruption or exception. Productivity directly contributes to the system performance. In our design, we would like to maximize productivity, while keeping the humans and robots safe. Any injury or damage should be avoided.

To maximize the productivity while maintaining safety, we use a weighted function to describe the overall award from the decisions. A policy with immediate reward is described as in:

$$Q_\pi(s, a) = E\{r_{t+1}|S_t = s, a_t = a, \pi\} \tag{6.3}$$

where s is the state, r is the reward, a is an action, π is a policy, and t is timing step. The reward r is computed as:

$$r_{t+1} = e^{||d-d_0||} * P + e^{-||d-d_0||} * S \qquad (6.4)$$

where P means productivity actions, and S means safety actions, d is the distance between a human and the TrayBot and d_o is a pre-defined threshold distance. Both P and S are binary variables, where value 1 means the robot decides to take the corresponding action, and 0 otherwise. P and S cannot be equal at the same time, i.e., the robot will not perform manipulation while taking the safety measures. In our design, safety task is of the highest priority and can override any manipulation tasks when required. This decision is made by maximizing the reward from equation Equ. 6.4.

Intuitively, when the distance between the robot and a human operator is smaller than a threshold d_0, the second term of Equ. 6.4 becomes negatively large. Then safety action will be taken (i.e. $S = 1$) to maximize $r_{(t+1)}$. If the distance is larger than d_0, the second term is also very small, then no safety action needs to be taken (i.e., S=0).

6.3.4 *Action*

Four safety regions are used in our system including *Safe, Caution, Danger*, and *Emergency* Stop. These regions are roughly correlated to the distance between the human and the TrayBot.

Using the positions of the tracked human in the environment and the pre-defined regions for different levels of safety, the decision-making module can trigger the Safety task to send out corresponding alarm signals. The Baxter will lift the right arm when a nurse is in the Danger zone and lift two arms when it is required to send out STOP signal.

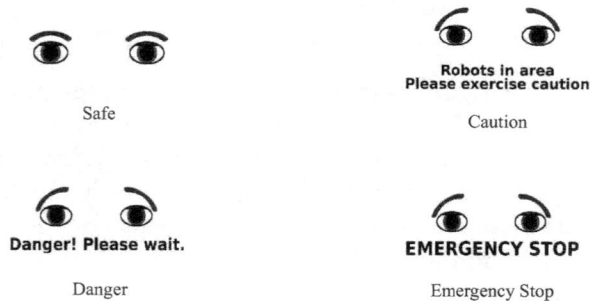

Safe

**Robots in area
Please exercise caution**

Caution

Danger! Please wait.

Danger

EMERGENCY STOP

Emergency Stop

Fig. 6.6   Facial expressions and texts displayed by Baxter and their corresponding safety regions.

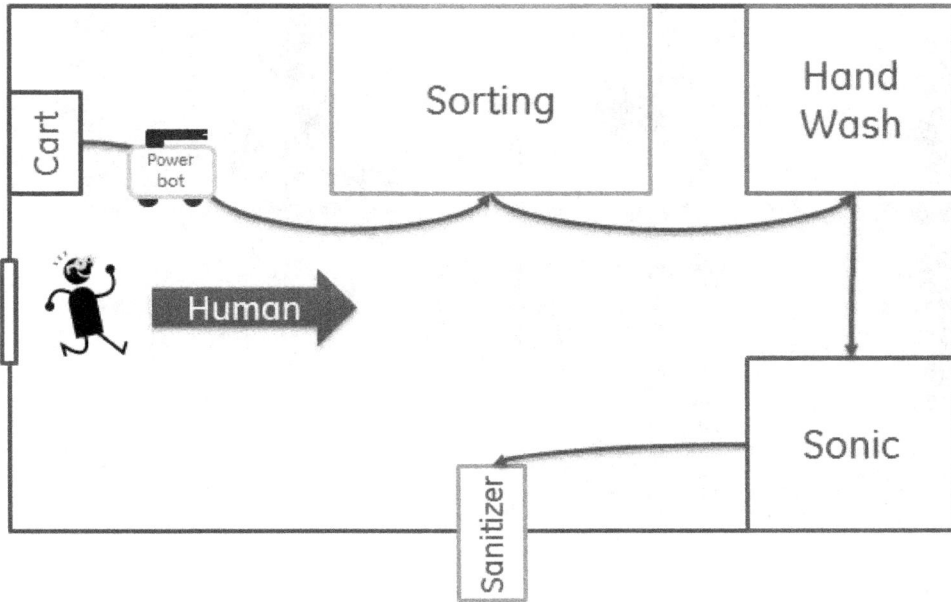

Fig. 6.7 Illustration of our experimental setup.

Additionally, Baxter's screen can show different facial expressions with texts for displaying warnings to the nurses who are working in the environment (Fig. 6.6. When a nurse is in different safety regions around the mobile robot, the Baxter will display different messages such as "Danger! Please wait" or "EMERGENCEY STOP".

6.4 Experiments and Results

Fig. 6.7 displays the experimental setup used to test our approach. When the TrayBot and the Baxter are working, a nurse enters the environment. The nurse will work in the environment together with TrayBot and Baxter to perform various tasks such as manual washing and disinfecting the dirty surgical instruments. When the nurse work at different working locations, his/her location is dynamic. The objective of our approach is to guarantee the safety of the human, which requires the Baxter send out corresponding alarm signals while the human works at different locations. Since this is a system integration level implementation, we only test the functional performance of our developed system. The quantitative results largely rely on different pieces in the system.

Fig. 6.8 is a photo showing how our method works. The Baxter monitors the environment using the Kinect sensor mounted on its head.

Fig. 6.9 displays a typical example of the various responses from the Baxter

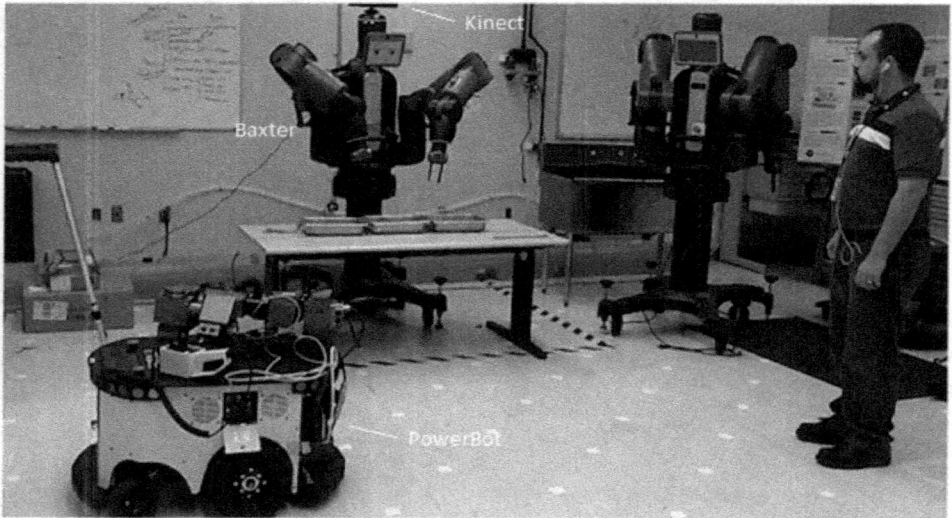

Fig. 6.8　Photo of our experimental setup.

when a human is already or is predicted to be in different safety zones. From the experimental results, we can see that the Baxter robot can correctly distinguish the current situation of the human in the environment, display corresponding image on the screen, and use its arms to send out corresponding signals.

The response time depends on the processing time of the Kinect sensor. The frame rate for Kinect sensor is related to the resolution of the images. The fastest rate is 30Hz. The control rate of the head is 1Hz. The control rate of the joint is also around 1Hz. That means, if we use Baxter's head and arm to send out safety signals, the response time is around 1100 ms. However, if we use other methods (e.g. sound alarms), it can largely reduce the response time to around 50ms. No matter what method we use, the response time is satisfactory unless somebody purposely runs very fast in the working room.

6.5　Conclusion and Future Work

This chapter proposes an integrated system for human-robot collaboration. The system is implemented using perception, recognition, reasoning, decision-making, and action. A vision-based sensory component is used for Baxter to monitor the environment and provide safety signals for humans. Experimental results demonstrate that our approach is effective in dealing with practical situations. In our experiments, we use one single mobile TrayBot. In the future, we will construct a dynamic environment where several mobile robots work collaboratively. In such a scenario, the reasoning and decision making process will be more complex. Currently, we only implemented a simple human detection-based system. In the future, we plan

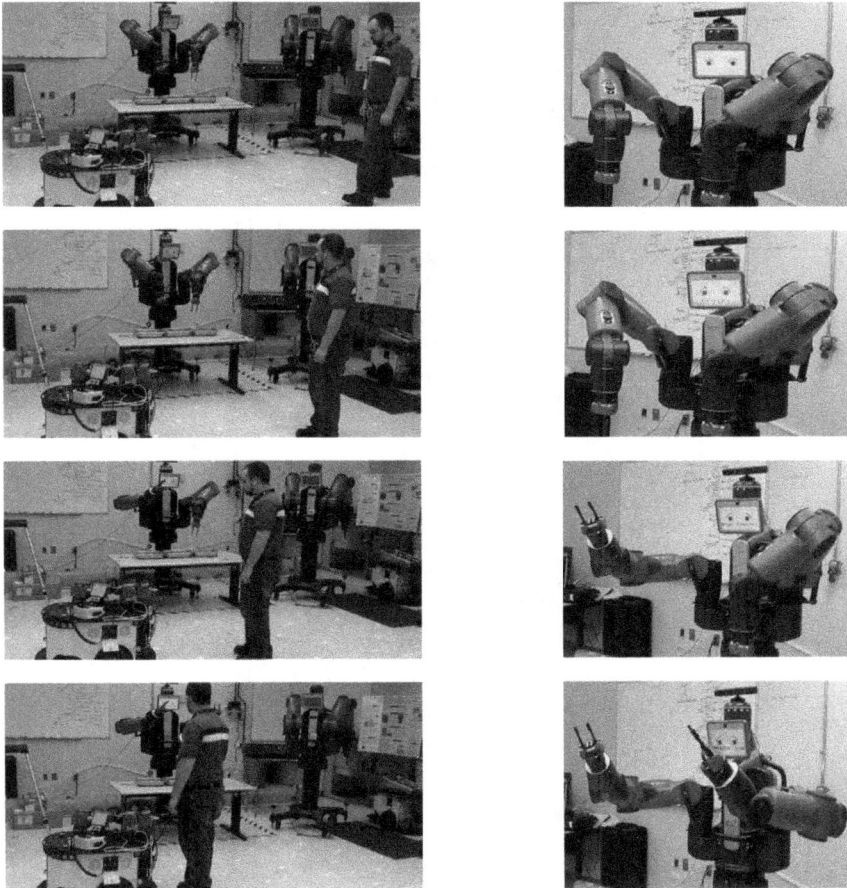

Fig. 6.9 Experiments results showing different response by Baxter.

to incorporate human action/gesture recognition in our system. Action/gesture recognition results can provide much more information for robots to analyze and predict human activities in the environment.

Chapter 7

Demonstration at VA

After developing all the technologies discussed in the previous chapters, we moved the robots to Orlando and demonstrated the prototype system in the VA hospital there. This chapter details the demonstration results and some of the challenges encountered by the team during the demonstration.

7.1 Demonstration Scope

The goal of the Integrated Automated Perioperative System Demo was to demonstrate to the VA sterile processing services (SPS) team the ability of integrated technologies to automate sterile processing facility. During the time of project proposal, we considered a comprehensive list of technologies we thought that can help achieve the goal of automated sterile processing. Fig. 7.1 specifies the different technologies being considered for each step in the automated solution. The list of technologies being proposed include:

- **TUG robot** for transporting carts between various parts of the hospital.
- **Robotray** for loading and unloading sterile kits onto carts.
- **Mobile robots** for moving kits through the sterilization process (autoclave, inventory, etc.) and delivering kits to the OR.
- **Fixed robotic arm** for sorting surgical implements and building kits.
- **Auto-ID technologies** such as 1D and 2D barcodes and radio frequency identification (RFID) for uniquely and accurately identifying and tracking implements and kits throughout the perioperative process.
- **Optical recognition** for identifying instruments for picking from a tray.
- **Conveyor system** for routing the surgical instrument kits to the proper autoclave for sterile processing and then to the proper inventory shelf for storage until needed.

Once the project started, we used an Agile development process which emphasized early feedback and the ability to accommodate evolving requirements quickly. The Agile development process allowed us to prototype and test multiple solutions quickly and change or pivot around them as appropriate. We learned through our

	Dirty Side		Clean Side						Hospital Corridors	
	Unload, count, rinse	Ultrasound	Wash / Disinfect	Inspect	Count	Sort	Pack	Sterilize	Inventory	Delivery
TUG Robot	✓									✓
Robotray	✓								✓	✓
Mobile Robot		✓						✓	✓	✓
Fixed Robotic Arm		✓		✓	✓	✓	✓	✓	✓	
Auto-ID	✓	✓	✓	✓	✓	✓	✓	✓	✓	✓
Optical Recognition		✓	✓	✓	✓	✓	✓	✓	✓	✓
Conveyor		✓	✓	✓		✓	✓	✓	✓	

Fig. 7.1   Considered options for the automated process.

interviews with several sterile processing centers that several pieces of the system were already automated at different facilities so we did not concentrate on these steps in the process. These steps included:

- **Autoclaves** Little Rock VA hospital has autoclaves on runners similar to rail tracks. When the rack is loaded, the SPS worker pushes a button and the autoclave doors open, the rack enters the autoclave automatically and the doors close until the cycle is complete. Then the doors automatically open again and the rack exits the autoclaves on its own.
- **Washer** - At the San Diego facility the washer racks are labeled with barcodes. When the rack is full, it moves on a conveyor to the washer, the barcode is read automatically and the controls on the washer are set to the proper setting according to that contents in the rack.
- **Sonicator** - The Orlando and San Diego facilities have sonicators that automatically raise and lower themselves by simply touching the front of the sonicator.

We also received feedback from the VA SPS team: 1. the team decided that they would not take people out of the inspection aspect of the SPS. 2. RFID is not a high priority due to the ongoing RLTS (Real Time Location System) efforts by the VA.

In addition to the interviews and feedback, we also made a few changes to our technology plan due to problem identified by early trial and error. For example, template based optical recognition algorithms are not good enough to identify a single instrument in a pile and a 2-fingered end effector could not pick up very small instrument, etc.

Based all these feedback and changes, we focused our demo on areas that could be automated and would have the greatest impact. These included:

(1) Validation of instruments returning from the OR to eliminate human error reading and writing numbers; sorting these instruments based on their types to facilitate manual cleaning.

(2) Moving instrument trays throughout the process to eliminate ergonomic issues in the workplace.

(3) Rebuilding kits to remove human error.

(4) Integration of machines and sensors to the system architecture to demonstrate the ability to interface with existing equipment such as the autoclaves, sonicators and sanitizers.

To this end, we used a subset of instruments, kit sizes and containers to develop the proof-of-concept.

7.2 Demonstration Technologies

In the following section, we will highlight the key technologies, their limitations, and associated reliability analysis for each of the key focus areas described above in the context of the system demonstration.

7.2.1 *Validation of Instruments Returning from the OR*

Technologies demonstrated:

- Robotics - TrayBot and Baxter
- Auto-ID - 2D Data Matrix
- Computer Vision - Instrument Singulation
- Mechatronics - Electromagnetic End Effector
- Integrated System Software Architecture

7.2.1.1 *Demonstrated Scenario*

Instrument trays are retrieved from a cart and delivered to the working table of Baxter robot by the TrayBot (Chapter 3). The instruments are in a pile in the tray. The computer vision algorithm determines which instrument is most likely on top and chooses the best location for the end effector to pick up the instrument based on the relative positions between instruments (Chapter 4). The computer vision algorithm then computes the XY coordinates of the pickup location on the working table and conveys these coordinates to the Baxter.

Baxter was outfitted with a custom designed electromagnetic end effector, which can be damped in 2 directions to ensure good contact between the magnet and the instrument, even when the instrument is not on a flat surface (Chapter 5). The end effector is also equipped with a force feedback sensor that informs Baxter when good contact is made with the surgical instrument. The end effector is integrated with Baxter using an Arduino® I/O board.

Baxter picks up the instrument on top as instructed by the computer vision algorithm and places the instrument into one of three trays based on the ID of the instrument. In the demonstration scenario, two of the trays require a different sanitization cycle and the third tray requires human inspection. Baxter is a collaborative robot and is aware of people that are in his workspace.

When the system determines there are no more instruments for sorting, the computer vision module sends a message to Baxter that the job is complete and then Baxter sends a message to the integrated system that this step was complete. The system then sends a message to the TrayBot to pick up the trays and deliver them to the next location.

7.2.1.2　*Limitations*

There are a few limitations with the current proof-of-concept.

Camera: We use a Nikon® D5200 SLR camera. Its field of view was limited to an approximate 10x12 inch rectangle in order to read the 2x2mm data matrix in the tray. This in turn limits the number of instruments in the space. The current algorithm analysis takes between 10 and 12 seconds per instrument. This time is unacceptable for commercialization purposes.

To accommodate this limitation, a camera with a higher resolution or multiple cameras can be utilized. The camera and its housing would also have to be improved to ensure it is able to be cleaned easily and certified for use in a SPS.

Baxter: Baxter is a first generation collaborative robot and has several limitations including payload (i.e., Baxter can only pick up objects less than 5 pounds). This limits the instruments we could use, the size of the tray and the number of instruments in the tray.

To address this, other commercial arms shall be evaluated. Another option would be to replace this robot station with a conveyor and 2D Data Matrix reader, similar to the solution of PenelopeCS™ [LaSelle (2011)].

2D Data Matrix: 2D Data Matrix ID stickers are used to identify instruments. We place the ID stickers on the optimal position on flat instruments. However, the IDs will have to be tested on round instruments for ID reading readability on a curved surface.

End effector: The end effector used in the demonstration is a prototype. It works well on flat instrument types where the surface of instrument and that of the magnet would have good contact. It has not been tested on circular instruments. Since the magnet has a diameter of one inch, when instruments are closely positioned it will sometimes pick up two instruments at the same time.

This limitation can be addressed in several ways. First, multiple end effectors may be required to pick up instruments of different shape and sizes. By comparing images of the tray, the system can determine whether one or more instruments are picked up and when one is dropped. In an instance where the system is unable to determine a method of grasping, the robot could reach out to a human teammate for assistance.

Integrated System Software Architecture: The system's architecture currently integrates to the VA's VistA system to demonstrate reporting capabilities. For the proof-of-concept, the system does not pull actual tray contents from the existing VistA system. Otherwise, the system can easily validate the list of instruments by reading the barcode IDs.

7.2.1.3 *Analytics and Reliability*

The Baxter robot was tested at the GE Global Research Center where the instruments were randomly placed into a tray for singulation. At the Community Living Center (CLC) in Orlando, effort was made to ensure consistency and best placement of the instruments to obtain 99-100% success rate for Baxter so that the proof-of-concept runs smoothly without human intervention.

Errors: All defects can be characterized into 3 types:

- Computer vision error - the top instrument is not identified by the algorithm
- Mechanical error - the gripper does not pick up the instrument the algorithm identified as the one on top or it picks up more than one instruments
- System error - all others such as, the gripper hits the side of the tray, etc.

Experimental Runs: The experiment data of Baxter is shown in Fig. 7.2. Run 1 and 2 were completed at GE Global Research (GRC) with 15 instruments placed in a random pile in the tray. Runs 3-9 were completed at Orlando CLC (Fla) on a subset of instruments to meet 99% success rate to ensure a smooth demo in Orlando.

After run 3 and before Run 4, it was observed that there was a bias between the targeted picking-up location and the actual picking-up location executed by Baxter. An offset was added for the algorithm to pick up slightly to the right of center for the Baxter end effector. This increased the success rate of Baxter from 83% to 96% on a subset of instruments. This indicates a calibration of Baxter can be improved.

After run 7, we arranged 6 instruments in optimal position for Baxter. This served 2 purposes: it shortened the amount of time of the proof-of-concept demo and it increased its success rate to 99%.

7.2.2 *Moving Instrument Trays Throughout the Process*

Technologies demonstrated:

- Robotics - Adept® PowerBot and Schunk® Arm
- Auto-ID - Fiducial marker (Chili tags)
- Computer Vision - simultaneous Localization and Mapping (SLAM)
- Mechatronics - Mechanical end effector and tray fixture
- Integrated System Software Architecture

	Baxter								
	GRC		Fla						
Run	1	2	3	4	5	6	7	8	9
# of Opp	120	156	12	24	60	90	30	54	102
Defects	34	35	2	1	1	1	0	0	1
% Accuracy	73	76	83	96	98	99	100	100	99

Fig. 7.2   Experimental Runs using Baxter

7.2.2.1 *Demonstrated Scenario*

Instruments are delivered to the SPS by a human operator in a tray on a cart. The instrument tray has a custom designed fixture attached to it. This allows the TrayBot to pick up the tray and keep it level as it is moved from station to station.

TrayBot is built using an Adept® mobile robot and completed with a Schunk® arm. The Adept® PowerBot is a mobile research robot. It is equipped with laser, sonar, gyroscope and odometer. The robot uses wheel odometry to estimate its position from the wheel rotation. The SICK® laser scanner located on the front of the robot is then used for more precise mapping and localization. In the demonstration, each processing step (e.g., Baxter table, sink, sonicator, etc.) is given a Cartesian coordinate associating it as a waypoint that the integrated system architecture can direct the TrayBot to move to. Each time TrayBot is given a direction to move to the next process step, it uses the Simultaneous Localization and Mapping (SLAM) algorithm to estimate its current location in the room and then move to the waypoint specified by the system to complete the next step in the process.

The TrayBot is equipped with a seven degrees of freedom (DOF) Schunk® arm. The end effector on the arm fits to the tray fixture to pick up the tray and keep it level as it moves from one processing position to the next. The TrayBot moves to a waypoint and then searches for a fiducial marker on the tray fixture to locate the correct tray using a camera mounted six inches above the gripper. The TrayBot uses a M-step searching strategy that can cover the entire working area of the table. If the desired ID of the tray is not found, the TrayBot generates a signal to notify human operators the task has failed. If the desired ID is found, the TrayBot picks up the tray and moves the tray from the cart to Baxter's working table. Later the TrayBot picks up and moves the tray from Baxter to the sinks for manual washing and inspection, from the sinks to the sonicator and from the sonicator to the sanitizer.

7.2.2.2 *Limitations*

Adept® Mobile Robot: As a research robot, the Adept® mobile PowerBot would need to be reconfigured with just the sensor technology needed for this specific application. The exterior should be redesigned so it is completely enclosed and easily cleaned and sanitized. The stainless steel fixtures in the SPS facility may interfere with the laser mapping.

Schunk® Arm: The 7-DOF arm is an overkill for picking up and moving the trays. A 5-DOF arm should be able to perform the same task with lower cost. The Schunk® arm can hold up to 20 pounds but not at its completely extended position. The Schunk® arm is meant to be modular; therefore it is designed with the electronics wiring to be on the outside of the robotic arm for easy configuration. This however, puts the system at risk if the wires catch on things at any point.

To address this limitation, we shall consider alternative collaborative robots such as the UR10 [Universal Robotics (2018)]. This arm is collaborative, can have a greater payload and designed to be more robust, electronically, than the Schunk® arm.

Mechanical End Effector and Fixture: The end effector and tray fixture work well to hold the tray in a level position. To address concern about its size, tests should be completed to determine the minimal footprint needed to hold a 27 pound tray of instruments. A visual fiducial tag (e.g., bar codes) already used by the VA Real Time Location System should be used to replace the Chilitags.

7.2.2.3 *Analytics and Reliability*

The TrayBot has been tested at the Orlando CLC and proven to be reliable time after time. During system testing, 25 runs were conducted requiring the TrayBpt to move 9 times each run for a total of 225 location changes. Only 1 error occurred: Traybot simply would not move. This occurred after 8 hours of continuous testing and no apparent reason could be found. The team rebooted the TrayBot and the system and it continued to work. This equates to 99.6% success rate.

7.2.3 *Rebuilding of Surgical Kits*

Technologies demonstrated:

- Robotics - Adept® Stationary Clean Room Certified Viper Arm
- Auto-ID - 2D Data Matrix
- Computer Vision - Instrument Singulation
- Mechatronics - Electromagnetic End Effector
- Integrated System Software Architecture

7.2.3.1 *Demonstrated Scenario*

In the demonstration, the instruments are delivered to the working table of the Adept® arm after the sanitation step by a SPS nurse in the process. The instruments are in a random pile in a tray. The same instrument singulation algorithm used by Baxter is used for the Adept® Viper arm. The computer vision algorithm determines which instrument is most likely on top and chooses the best location for the end effector to pick up the instrument.

The Adept® Viper arm is outfitted with the same type of custom designed electromagnetic end effector as Baxter. The end effector is also equipped with a force feedback sensor that informs the Viper arm when it has made contact with the instrument. The Adept® controller is programmed to control the end effector force. Before releasing the instrument in the desired location in the surgical kit, the controller quickly oscillates the electromagnetic current. This allows the system to remove any residual magnetism from the instrument. The Viper arm picks up the instrument on top and precisely places the instrument into one of 2 trays based on the ID and the surgical kit it is instructed to build. In the demonstration, the three trays of instruments separated by Baxter are rebuilt into two instrument kits.

The Viper arm is a commercially available, extremely precise robotic arm (0.01mm precision vs. 5mm precision for Baxter). It is unaware of people in its surroundings and moves at speeds up to 0.8m/s in the proof-of-concept. The Viper arm requires to have additional safety features such as an enclosure to protect workers from harm when it is in full automation mode.

When the computer vision algorithm determines there are no more instruments for sorting, it sends a message to the Viper arm that the job is complete and then the Adept® Controller sends a message to the integrated system that the kit-building step is complete. The system then sent a message to the M2M conveyor system to move the trays to the next step.

7.2.3.2 *Limitations*

The overhead camera, 2D Data Matrix IDs, and electromagnetic end effector used on the clean side is the same as the dirty side, so the limitations described in Section 7.2.1.2 are also present with clean side operation.

7.2.3.3 *Analytics and Reliability*

The Adept® Viper arm was tested at the GE Global Research Center where the instruments were randomly placed into a tray for singulation. At the Community Living Center (CLC) in Orlando, effort was made to ensure consistency and best placement of the instruments to obtain 99-100% success rate for Adept® so that the proof-of-concept runs smoothly without human intervention.

Experimental Runs: experiment data of Adept stationary arm is shown in Fig. 7.3. Run 1 and 2 were completed at GE Global Research (GRC) with 15

Adept								
	GRC		Fla					
Run	1	2	3	4	5	6	7	8	9
# of Opp	118	60	12	24	60	90	30	54	102
Defects	6	9	2	2	5	6	1	1	1
% Accuracy	95	85	83	92	92	93	97	98	99

Fig. 7.3   Experimental runs using Adept.

instruments placed in a random pile in the tray. Runs 3-9 were completed at Orlando CLC (Fla) on a subset of instruments to meet 99% success rate to ensure a smooth demo in Orlando.

After run 6, an instrument (single use Pakistan instrument - low grade SS) is removed since it is responsible for 50% of the errors.

After run 8 we arranged instruments in optimal position for Adept. This increased its success rate to 99%.

7.2.4 *Machine and Sensor Integration*

Technologies demonstrated:

- Hardware - conveyor, IR sensors, automatic AC indicator dispenser
- Integrated System Software Architecture

7.2.4.1 *Demonstrated Scenario*

After the Adept® Viper arm rebuild the surgical instrument kits, the Adept® Controller sends a message to the integrated system architecture to turn on the conveyor belt. The conveyor moves the surgical kits to the station where it passes an IR sensor. When trigger, the sensor is configured to turn the conveyor off and turn on an automatic dispenser to dispense the autoclave indicator into the completed surgical kit. A human SPS operator then picks up the surgical kit and moves it to the inspection station to validate the kit. After inspection, the operator places the filter paper inside the kit and put the lid on the kit. When the human operator removes the kit from the conveyor, the conveyor will be reactivated again and moves the next surgical kit to the indicator dispenser.

7.2.4.2 *Limitations*

This step in the demonstration is a very robust display of M2M technology. Sensors and conveyor technologies can be used in several areas of the sterile processing to reduce cost and increase reliability.

7.3 Final Thoughts

The different pieces of technologies are highly modular and can be integrated together using our software architecture. This allows us to implement an automated sterile processing system using different configurations. In this section, two scenarios will be presented and the technology to commercialize will be discussed. In the first scenario, humans and robots collaboratively working in the SPS together. Second scenario is a lights out operation with no humans in the operation. The commercialization requirements are based on processing 20,000 instruments in 24 hours.

7.3.1 *Human-Robot Collaboration*

7.3.1.1 *Option 1*

In this current scenario, human operator delivers the used instruments from the OR to the SPS where a mobile robot moves them throughout the process on the dirty side and the clean side. Baxter sorts the instruments on the dirty side and Adept® remakes the kits on the clean side.

To commercialize, the computer vision algorithm has to be further developed to process images within 2 seconds.

7.3.1.2 *Option 2*

One option is that we can eliminate the computer vision algorithm from Baxter and Adept and replace it with a bar code reader. On the dirty side of the process, this would eliminate Baxter from the process and replace Baxter with a conveyor to move the instruments over a bar code reader then to a sorter that will move instruments to the sinks for inspection and washing.

On the clean side, a human operator places the instruments on a conveyor, which moves the instruments past a bar code reader to inform the Adept® arm which instrument is present and the Adept® arm can retrieve it from the conveyor to build the kit.

To commercialize, a conveyor based sorting system has to be developed.

7.3.2 *Lights Out*

The second scenario removes all human operators from the process. Instruments would be delivered from the OR to the SPS using an unmanned ground vehicle

(UGV). The UGV would place the contents of the returned container onto a gently shaking conveyor moving over small obstacles, which would align the instruments and thin the pile out as the instruments moved down the conveyor. At the end of the conveyor, the instruments would pass over a bar code reader where the IDs would be compared to a list of expected instruments provided by the system. The instruments would be sorted into bins that would be fed into automatic washers and sonicators, then to the sanitizer. The sanitizer would set the proper cycle for the contents using data from the integrated system.

The UGV would guide itself to the cart cleaner for cleaning and then to a queue until needed for the next delivery.

On the clean side, the sanitizer racks would gently unload the instruments onto a similar gently shaking conveyor with obstacles that would align the instruments and direct them over a bar code reader. The IDs would be sent to an event manager that would direct the instrument to an inspection station. The inspection station would require development of fixtures to possibly open and close an instrument, to increase or decrease available light, etc. Additional computer vision algorithm would need to be developed for automatic inspection. The instruments would pass from the inspection station to the build stations.

Each instrument passing inspection would be diverted to a particular stationary robot so all the required instruments are fed to the robot so it can build the kit as optimally as possible. For instance, if it is a two layer kit, the robot would build the bottom layer first. The robot should have all the instruments for that kit in its range of motion before starting to build the kit. To effectively handle multiple types of instruments would require multiple end effectors so each robot would have to have a quick changing end effector station depending on the instrument it was currently picking and placing. Also, multiple fixtures would be required depending on the instrument. Fixtures would be needed for things such as stringers and sharps. The build station should also have automatic filter paper placement, biological indicator addition and lid closure capabilities.

After the kits are built, conveyors could move the containers onto an autoclave rack that is integrated to an automated autoclave system. The rack records container ID, autoclave ID, temperature and pressure, date and time stamps and communicates this directly to the event manager. The containers are autoclaved and automatically unloaded after drying and cooling. The rack can be moved to central inventory where the surgical kits stay on the rack until needed in the OR. The UGV could retrieve containers as needed based on the scheduling of the OR and deliver the sterile containers to the OR.

Bibliography

2D Technology Group (2018). 2dtg — barcode decoding, brand protection, dpm scanners, rugged mobile computers, https://www.2dtg.com/.

Adept Mobilerobots (2016). PowerBot, Retrieved from URL http://www.mobilerobots.com/Accessories/PowerBotArm.aspx/.

Aethon (2018). Tug robots in healthcare, "http://www.aethon.com/tug/tughealthcare/.

Albus, J. S. and Barbera, A. J. (2005). Rcs: A cognitive architecture for intelligent multi-agent systems, *Annual Reviews in Control* **29**, 1, pp. 87 – 99.

Alefs, B., Eschemann, G., Ramoser, H., and Beleznai, C. (2007). Road sign detection from edge orientation histograms, in *2007 IEEE Intelligent Vehicles Symposium*, pp. 993–998.

Anderson, J. R. and Lebiere, C. J. (eds.) (1998). *The Atomic Components of Thought* (Lawrence Erlbaum Associates, Mahwah, NJ), ISBN 978-0-8058-2816-0.

Asimov, I. (2004). *I, robot*, Vol. 1 (Spectra).

Bast, P., Popovic, A., Wu, T., Heger, S., Engelhardt, M., Lauer, W., Radermacher, K., and Schmieder, K. (2006). Robot and computer-assisted craniotomy: resection planning, implant modelling and robot safety, *The International Journal of Medical Robotics and Computer Assisted Surgery* **2**, 2, pp. 168–178.

Bonnard, Q., Lemaignan, S., Zufferey, G., Mazzei, A., Cuendet, S., Li, N., Özgür, A., and Dillenbourg, P. (2013). Chilitags 2: Robust fiducial markers for augmented reality and robotics. http://chili.epfl.ch/software.

Brooks, R. (1986). A robust layered control system for a mobile robot, *IEEE Journal on Robotics and Automation* **2**, 1, pp. 14–23.

Causey, G. C. and Quinn, R. D. (1998). Gripper design guidelines for modular manufacturing, in *Proceedings. 1998 IEEE International Conference on Robotics and Automation (Cat. No.98CH36146)*, Vol. 2, pp. 1453–1458 vol.2.

Censitrac (2018). The leader in surgical asst management: Censis technologies, http://www.censis.net/.

Chitta, S., Jones, E. G., Ciocarlie, M., and Hsiao, K. (2012). Mobile manipulation in unstructured environments: Perception, planning, and execution, *IEEE Robotics Automation Magazine* **19**, 2, pp. 58–71.

Choi, C., Taguchi, Y., Tuzel, O., Liu, M. Y., and Ramalingam, S. (2012). Voting-based pose estimation for robotic assembly using a 3d sensor, in *2012 IEEE International Conference on Robotics and Automation*, pp. 1724–1731.

Choset, H. M. (2005). *Principles of robot motion: theory, algorithms, and implementation* (MIT press).

Collet, A., Martinez, M., and Srinivasa, S. S. (2011). The moped framework: Object recognition and pose estimation for manipulation, *The International Journal of Robotics Research* **30**, 10, pp. 1284–1306.

Dalal, N. and Triggs, B. (2005). Histograms of oriented gradients for human detection, in *2005 IEEE Computer Society Conference on Computer Vision and Pattern Recognition (CVPR'05)*, Vol. 1, pp. 886–893 vol. 1.

DFKI (2018). AILA mobile dual-arm-manipulation, Retrieved from URL `http://robotik.dfki-bremen.de/en/research/robot-systems/aila.html/`.

DLR (2016). Rollin' Justin, Retrieved from URL `http://www.dlr.de/rm/en/desktopdefault.aspx/tabid-5471/8991_read-16694/`.

Dollar, A. M. and Howe, R. D. (2010). The highly adaptive sdm hand: Design and performance evaluation, *The international journal of robotics research* **29**, 5, pp. 585–597.

Fryman, J. and Matthias, B. (2012). Safety of industrial robots: From conventional to collaborative applications, in *ROBOTIK 2012; 7th German Conference on Robotics*, pp. 1–5.

Gobet, F., Lane, P., Croker, S., Cheng, P., Jones, G., Oliver, I., and Pine, J. (2001). Chunking mechanisms in human learning, .

Guizzo, E. and Ackerman, E. (2012). How rethink robotics built its new baxter robot worker, *IEEE spectrum* , p. 18.

Haddadin, S., Albu-Schäffer, A., and Hirzinger, G. (2009). Requirements for safe robots: Measurements, analysis and new insights, *The International Journal of Robotics Research* **28**, 11-12, pp. 1507–1527.

Hayashibe, M., Suzuki, N., and Nakamura, Y. (2006). Laser-scan endoscope system for intraoperative geometry acquisition and surgical robot safety management, *Medical Image Analysis* **10**, 4, pp. 509 – 519, special Issue on Functional Imaging and Modelling of the Heart (FIMH 2005).

Hsiao, E. and Hebert, M. (2012). Occlusion reasoning for object detection under arbitrary viewpoint, in *2012 IEEE Conference on Computer Vision and Pattern Recognition*, pp. 3146–3153.

ISO (2014). ISO 13482:2014 Robots and robotic devices - safety requirements for personal care robots, `https://www.iso.org/standard/53820.html`.

ISO (2016). ISO 7153-1:2016 standard, surgical instruments materials part 1: Metals, `https://www.iso.org/standard/66850.html`.

Kam, M., Zhu, X., and Kalata, P. (1997). Sensor fusion for mobile robot navigation, *Proceedings of the IEEE* **85**, 1, pp. 108–119.

Key Surgical (2018). Key surgical — sterile processing products and o.r. supplies, Retrieved from URL `http://www.keysurgical.com/`.

Khatib, O. (1986). Real-time obstacle avoidance for manipulators and mobile robots, *The international journal of robotics research* **5**, 1, pp. 90–98.

Kieras, D. E. and Meyer, D. E. (1997). An overview of the epic architecture for cognition and performance with application to human-computer interaction, *Human-Computer Interaction* **12**, 4, pp. 391–438.

Klein, G. and Murray, D. (2007). Parallel tracking and mapping for small ar workspaces, in *2007 6th IEEE and ACM International Symposium on Mixed and Augmented Reality*, pp. 225–234.

Kwak, S., Nam, W., Han, B., and Han, J. H. (2011). Learning occlusion with likelihoods for visual tracking, in *2011 International Conference on Computer Vision*, pp. 1551–1558.

LaSelle,   R.   (2011).   Automating sterile supply departments protects patients, "`https://www.healthmgttech.com/automating-sterile-supply-departments-protects-patients.php`.

Lehman, J. F., Laird, J., and Rosenbloom, P. (1996). A gentle introduction to soar, an architecture for human cognition, in S. Sternberg and D. Scarborough (eds.), *Invitation to Cognitive Science: Methods, Models, and Conceptual Issues*, Vol. 4 (MIT Press).

Leonard, J. J. and Durrant-Whyte, H. F. (1991). Simultaneous map building and localization for an autonomous mobile robot, in *Intelligent Robots and Systems '91. 'Intelligence for Mechanical Systems, Proceedings IROS '91. IEEE/RSJ International Workshop on*, Vol. 3, pp. 1442–1447.

Lewis, F. L., Dawson, D. M., and Abdallah, C. T. (2003). *Robot manipulator control: theory and practice* (CRC Press).

Liu, M.-Y., Tuzel, O., Veeraraghavan, A., Taguchi, Y., Marks, T. K., and Chellappa, R. (2012). Fast object localization and pose estimation in heavy clutter for robotic bin picking, *The International Journal of Robotics Research* **31**, 8, pp. 951–973.

Mur-Artal, R., Montiel, J. M. M., and Tards, J. D. (2015). Orb-slam: A versatile and accurate monocular slam system, *IEEE Transactions on Robotics* **31**, 5, pp. 1147–1163.

NASA Johnson Space Center (2016). Robonaut 2, Retrieved from URL `http://robonaut.jsc.nasa.gov`.

Nieuwenhuisen, M., Droeschel, D., Holz, D., Stckler, J., Berner, A., Li, J., Klein, R., and Behnke, S. (2013). Mobile bin picking with an anthropomorphic service robot, in *2013 IEEE International Conference on Robotics and Automation*, pp. 2327–2334.

Padois, V., Fourquet, J.-Y., and Chiron, P. (2007). Kinematic and dynamic model-based control of wheeled mobile manipulators: A unified framework for reactive approaches, *Robotica* **25**, 2, pp. 157–173.

Papazov, C., Haddadin, S., Parusel, S., Krieger, K., and Burschka, D. (2012). Rigid 3d geometry matching for grasping of known objects in cluttered scenes, *The International Journal of Robotics Research* **31**, 4, pp. 538–553.

Parmiggiani, A., Randazzo, M., Natale, L., and Metta, G. (2014). An alternative approach to robot safety, in *2014 IEEE/RSJ International Conference on Intelligent Robots and Systems*, pp. 484–489.

Pretto, A., Tonello, S., and Menegatti, E. (2013). Flexible 3d localization of planar objects for industrial bin-picking with monocamera vision system, in *2013 IEEE International Conference on Automation Science and Engineering (CASE)*, pp. 168–175.

Rahardja, K. and Kosaka, A. (1996). Vision-based bin-picking: recognition and localization of multiple complex objects using simple visual cues, in *Intelligent Robots and Systems '96, IROS 96, Proceedings of the 1996 IEEE/RSJ International Conference on*, Vol. 3, pp. 1448–1457 vol.3.

Reardon, C., Tan, H., Kannan, B., and DeRose, L. (2015). Towards safe robot-human collaboration systems using human pose detection, in *2015 IEEE International Conference on Technologies for Practical Robot Applications (TePRA)*, pp. 1–6.

Rethink Robotics (2018). Rethink robotics — smart collaborative robots — advanced automation technology, `http://www.rethinkrobotics.com/`.

Rodrigues, J. J., Kim, J. S., Furukawa, M., Xavier, J., Aguiar, P., and Kanade, T. (2012). 6d pose estimation of textureless shiny objects using random ferns for bin-picking, in *2012 IEEE/RSJ International Conference on Intelligent Robots and Systems*, pp. 3334–3341.

Rublee, E., Rabaud, V., Konolige, K., and Bradski, G. (2011). Orb: An efficient alternative to sift or surf, in *2011 International Conference on Computer Vision*, pp. 2564–2571.

Saito, T. and Ikeda, H. (2007). Development of normally closed type of magnetorheological clutch and its application to safe torque control system of human-collaborative robot,

Journal of Intelligent Material Systems and Structures **18**, 12, pp. 1181–1185.

Sam, R. and Nefti, S. (2008). Design and development of flexible robotic gripper for handling food products, in *2008 10th International Conference on Control, Automation, Robotics and Vision*, pp. 1684–1689.

Saxena, A., Driemeyer, J., and Ng, A. Y. (2008). Robotic grasping of novel objects using vision, *The International Journal of Robotics Research* **27**, 2, pp. 157–173.

Schneider, W. (1999). *Working Memory in a Multilevel Hybrid Connectionist Control Architecture (CAP2)* (Cambridge University Press), pp. 340–374, doi:10.1017/ CBO9781139174909.013.

Seraji, H. (1998). A unified approach to motion control of mobile manipulators, *The International Journal of Robotics Research* **17**, 2, pp. 107–118.

Shrobe, H., Winston, P., Tennenbaum, J., Shaftoe, P., Massaquoi, S., Robertson, P., Williams, B., Eslick, I., Rao, S., Coen, M., *et al.* (2006). Chip: A cognitive architecture for comprehensive human intelligence and performance, *Electronic Resource: http://www. darpa. mil/ipto/programs/bica/phase1. htm* , pp. 177–188.

Shroff, N., Taguchi, Y., Tuzel, O., Veeraraghavan, A., Ramalingam, S., and Okuda, H. (2011). Finding a needle in a specular haystack, in *2011 IEEE International Conference on Robotics and Automation*, pp. 5963–5970, doi:10.1109/ICRA.2011.5979857.

Srinivasa, S. S., Ferguson, D., Helfrich, C. J., Berenson, D., Collet, A., Diankov, R., Gallagher, G., Hollinger, G., Kuffner, J., and Weghe, M. V. (2010). HERB: a home exploring robotic butler, *Autonomous Robots* **28**, 1, pp. 5–20.

Sun, R. (2003). A tutorial on clarion 5.0, Tech. rep., Cognitive Science Department, Rensselaer Polytechnic Institute.

Tan, H. (2012). Implementation of a framework for imitation learning on a humanoid robot using a cognitive architecture, in *The Future of Humanoid Robots-Research and Applications* (InTech).

Tan, H. (2013). *Integration of Imitation Learning with Cognitive Control for a Humanoid Robot*, Ph.D. thesis, Vanderbilt University.

Tan, H. (2014). Imitation learning and behavior generation in a robot team, in *Distributed Autonomous Robotic Systems, Springer Tracts in Advanced Robotics*, Vol. 104 (Springer, Berlin, Heidelberg), pp. 423–434.

Tan, H., Holovashchenko, V., Mao, Y., Kannan, B., and DeRose, L. (2015a). Human-supervisory distributed robotic system architecture for healthcare operation automation, in *2015 IEEE International Conference on Systems, Man, and Cybernetics*, pp. 133–138.

Tan, H. and Liang, C. (2011). A conceptual cognitive architecture for robots to learn behaviors from demonstrations in robotic aid area, in *2011 Annual International Conference of the IEEE Engineering in Medicine and Biology Society*, pp. 1249–1252.

Tan, H., Liao, Q., and Zhou, Y. (2007). Design and qualitative analysis of the improved algorithm of motion track predictive control with flexible curve calculation for robot manipulator, in *Proceedings of 2007 International Conference on Intelligent Systems and Control*.

Tan, H., Mao, Y., Xu, Y., Kannan, B., Griffin, W. B., and DeRose, L. (2016). An integrated robotic system for transporting surgical tools in hospitals, in *2016 Annual IEEE Systems Conference (SysCon)*, pp. 1–8.

Tan, H., Xu, Y., Mao, Y., Tong, X., Griffin, W. B., Kannan, B., and DeRose, L. A. (2015b). An integrated vision-based robotic manipulation system for sorting surgical tools, in *2015 IEEE International Conference on Technologies for Practical Robot Applications (TePRA)*, pp. 1–6.

Universal Robotics (2018). Collaborative industrial robotic robot arms — cobots from universal robots, `http://www.universal-robots.com/`.

Wang, X., Han, T. X., and Yan, S. (2009). An hog-lbp human detector with partial occlusion handling, in *2009 IEEE 12th International Conference on Computer Vision*, pp. 32–39.

Willow Garage (2015). PR2 overview, Retrieved from URL `http://www.willowgarage.com/pages/pr2/overview`.

Winikoff, M. (2005). Jack^{TM} intelligent agents: an industrial strength platform. in R. H. Bordini, M. Dastani, J. Dix, and A. E. Fallah-Seghrouchni (eds.), *Multi-Agent Programming, Multiagent Systems, Artificial Societies, and Simulated Organizations*, Vol. 15 (Springer), ISBN 0-387-24568-5, pp. 175–193.

Xu, Y., Mao, Y., Tong, X., Tan, H., Griffin, W. B., Kannan, B., and DeRose, L. A. (2015). Robotic handling of surgical instruments in a cluttered tray, *IEEE Transactions on Automation Science and Engineering* **12**, 2, pp. 775–780.

Xu, Y., Tong, X., Mao, Y., Griffin, W. B., Kannan, B., and DeRose, L. A. (2014). A vision-guided robot manipulator for surgical instrument singulation in a cluttered environment, in *2014 IEEE International Conference on Robotics and Automation (ICRA)*, pp. 3517–3523.

Zhang, T. and Goldberg, K. (2001). Design of robot gripper jaws based on trapezoidal modules, in *Proceedings 2001 ICRA. IEEE International Conference on Robotics and Automation (Cat. No.01CH37164)*, Vol. 2, pp. 1065–1070 vol.2.

Zhang, Z. (2012). Microsoft kinect sensor and its effect, *IEEE MultiMedia* **19**, 2, pp. 4–10.

Index